The National Board for Certification in Occupational Therapy, Inc. (NBCOT®) is pleased to publish the Official Examination Study Guide for the CERTIFIED OCCUPATIONAL THERAPY ASSISTANT COTA® (COTA) Certification Examination. The occupational therapy content of this guide has been aligned to the examination test specifications of NBCOT's 2007 Practice Analysis Study. The results of this study were used to guide examination items that will subsequently be used on NBCOT certification examinations beginning January 2009.

The purpose of this study guide is to provide:

- a tool that will assist candidates in gaining an understanding of the certification process;
- examples of practice-focused multiple-choice items for the COTA; and
- a means to assist candidates with their test preparation.

The primary purpose for developing this study guide is to provide information to candidates that can be used to support and augment their overall examination preparation activities. By purchasing this guide, no inference should be made or assumed that by using this guide it ensures success on the certification examination.

The development of this guide, and most importantly the certification examination, would not have been possible without the professionalism and expertise of a dedicated legion of COTA and OCCUPATIONAL THERAPIST REGISTERED OTR® practitioners and educators who participated in NBCOT's item writing activities and/or on the Certification Examination Validation Committee (CEVC). The breadth and depth of the material in this guide would not have been possible without their participation.

Paul Grace, MS, CAE
President and Chief Executive Officer, NBCOT

NBCOT... serving the public interest

Contents

Appendices

Historically, regulation of the health professions in the United States began with a necessity to protect the public from the under-educated and under-trained professional. Over time, licensure, credentialing and certification have continued the tradition of protecting the public but have also increased their scope of activity to continuously improve the quality of practice in the profession.

Certification is a process by which key required competencies for practice are measured, and the professional is endorsed by a board of his/her peers (Barnhart, 1997). Earned certification means an individual has met a specified quality standard that reflects nationally-accepted practice principles and values (McClain, Richardson & Wyatt, 2004). The purpose of awarding the credential – CERTIFIED OCCUPATIONAL THERAPY ASSISTANT (COTA®) - is to identify for the public those persons who have demonstrated the knowledge and the skills necessary to provide occupational therapy assistant services. Certification has become the hallmark credential for professionals in a variety of industries, often serving as a benchmark for hiring and promotion (Microsoft, 2003). For more than 50 years, the COTA "mark" has been recognized by agencies, employers, payers, and consumers as viable symbols of quality educated and currently prepared practitioners.

The National Board for Certification in Occupational Therapy (NBCOT®) is a not-for-profit credentialing agency responsible for the development and implementation of policies related to the certification of occupational therapy practitioners in the United States. This independent national credentialing agency grants the COTA certification to eligible individuals. The primary mission of NBCOT is to "serve the public interest." NBCOT certification uses a formal process to grant a certification credential to an individual who: 1) meets academic and practice experience requirements; 2) successfully completes a comprehensive examination to assess knowledge and skills for practice; and 3) agrees to adhere to the NBCOT Candidate/Certificant Code of Conduct. Currently, 47 states, Guam, Puerto Rico and the District of Columbia require NBCOT initial certification for occupational therapy state regulation, e.g., licensing.

Overview and Purpose of the Study Guide

This study guide has five sections:

- ◘ Section 1 contains information about adult learning including thinking critically, learning as an adult, scheduling time for study, and controlling the study environment.

- ◘ Section 2 examines strategies for developing successful study habits such as using memory effectively, avoiding procrastination, and utilizing cooperative learning techniques.

- ◘ Section 3 considers general test-taking strategies including things to do before, during, and after the test, overcoming test anxiety, and guidelines for answering multiple-choice questions.

- ◘ Section 4 refers specifically to the NBCOT certification examination, including how NBCOT uses the results of practice analysis studies to guide test construction, and general administrative procedures specific to the NBCOT certification examination.

- ◼ Section 5 contains 100 multiple-choice COTA sample items representative of the domains and task areas found in the test blueprint. Although the items included in the study guide practice test are grouped by domain and task areas to illustrate the type of questions that may be representative of a particular domain, questions on the actual certification examination will not appear grouped by domain, but will be randomized. **None of the questions included in this study guide will appear on the NBCOT certification examination.** In addition to presenting sample items, this section also contains an answer key, a rationale for the correct response, an explanation of why the distractors are incorrect, and references for additional information.

- ◼ Appendix A contains a copy of the COTA Examination Readiness Tool, Appendix B includes a reference list, Appendix C provides a listing of standard abbreviations used on the certification examination, Appendix D includes interventions, service components, and settings commonly used on the certification examination, and Appendix E includes the 2007 Blueprint Specifications for the COTA validated domain, task, and knowledge statements.

This study guide should be used as only one tool in preparing to take the certification examination. The examination questions are designed to test the knowledge necessary for entry-level practice. Reviewing course materials, texts, and fieldwork experiences are other ways that candidates can prepare for the certification examination. This study guide will supplement preparation efforts by providing information on the testing process and the structure of the questions that are used on the NBCOT certification examination.

NBCOT does not administer, approve, or endorse review or preparatory courses for the certification examination. It is NBCOT's mission that the COTA certification examination is reflective of current entry-level certified occupational therapy assistant practice. Practice tests, available on NBCOT's website at *www.nbcot.org*, provide additional opportunities for test preparation. Certification examination review courses are advertised and available to candidates. However, these courses are not endorsed by NBCOT.

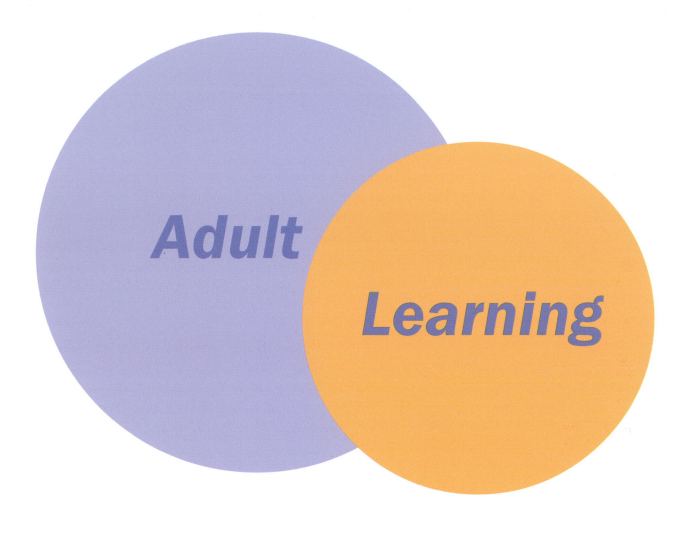

Thinking Critically

Learning to think critically is one of the most significant activities of adult life (Brookfield, 1987). Indeed, it can be argued that without critical thinking, the individual views the world through a single, isolated lens, with no awareness of how others view their actions, or respect for the way others behave or make decisions about their world. To think critically is to become open to alternative ways of looking at, and behaving in, the world. As Brookfield (1987) reminds us, it is through critical thinking that we learn to pay attention to the context in which we (and others) think, act, and behave.

Critical thinking should be a core skill for all successful occupational therapy practitioners. It is through critical thinking that the occupational therapy practitioner creates and recreates aspects of the client's life. Critical thinkers are innovators, concerned with the potential for improvement while at the same time, respecting diversity of values, behaviors, and structures that guide the client's world. Critical thinking entails continual questioning of assumptions and an ongoing appreciation of the context in which life occurs. For example, the occupational therapy practitioner will appreciate that a person who has recently become a wheelchair user will experience an array of thoughts and emotions associated with this newly acquired mobility device. The person may feel happy that this device is enabling them to gain access into their community. On the other hand, they may feel embarrassed, or frustrated for others to see that they are having to rely on a mobility device to do the things that they were previously able to do.

All occupational therapy entry-level curricula seek to develop critical thinking skills to prepare their students for successful future practice. However, the skill of critical thinking can also be used as an important strategy for studying and preparing to take high stakes examinations such as the NBCOT COTA certification examination. The following provides a framework of how to apply critical thinking to your studying routines:

1. *Define what it is that you want to learn.* You may be familiar with the anatomical implications of ulnar nerve palsy for example, but want to know more about how this impacts thumb mobility and the challenges posed by this condition for a homemaker caring for a young child. In this sense, you could use critical thinking to help you appreciate the perspective of this homemaker. Define your learning into simple phrases such as:

   - How does the impairment affect ability to button the baby's clothes?
   - How might this impact ability to carry out grooming tasks?
   - Would adaptations be needed to open packets of formula?

2. *Think about what you already know about the subject.* Critical thinking will help you to identify strengths and gaps in your knowledge. Tapping into your previous experiences from fieldwork, labs, case studies, and readings, will give you a foundation upon which to build your learning. It will also help you to identify any prejudices that may be coloring the way you are currently conducting your studying. For example, you may be reluctant to invest much time in considering how you might design a pre-vocational skills program for someone with a substance abuse disorder if you have an underlying prejudice about people who abuse alcohol. Addressing these prejudices will enable you to view situations with an open mind, and aid your studying and ongoing journey towards successful future practice.

3. *Identify resources.* Critical thinking is about recognizing and using all the resources that are available to you. In this sense, consider resources in the widest possible context, have an open mind. These are a few you may consider, expand on these and design your own list:

- People – professors, fieldwork educators, mentors, peer group, community members, case studies
- Materials – textbooks, journal readings, reflective journals, class notes, lab exercises, videos or DVDs
- Environments – fieldwork, community facilities, specialist clinics, adaptive workplaces, inpatient services

4. *Ask questions.* Use your critical thinking skills to enhance your understanding. Do you hold underlying beliefs about this disorder and is this influencing your studying? Does this author have prejudices about the information they are presenting? Is this professor telling you the full story about what it is like living with this disability? Continue to ask questions – why/what/how/if...

5. *Organize the information you have gathered.* Use your critical thinking skills to examine patterns and make connections across your learning. For example, you have reviewed your understanding about ulnar nerve palsy, talked to a certified occupational therapy assistant who has worked with people who have this condition, discussed ways this condition may affect household occupations with your peers, and identified possible intervention strategies to assist this condition.

6. *Demonstrate your knowledge.* Pulling all this information together, think of ways to demonstrate what you now know. Use lists, flowcharts, and summary statements to highlight key information. Discuss comparisons and similarities of disorders and strategies for overcoming occupational challenges. Write up a report with recommendations for treatment interventions.

> *Remember, have an open mind to enable you to gather resources to aid your learning. Group information together to increase understanding. Use critical thinking skills to enhance your studying.*

Learning as an Adult

Through your occupational therapy education, you will have identified that there are many different ways to learn information. You will also be familiar with evaluating and selecting the most appropriate learning strategy to meet the needs of the clients you are working with. You can use the same strategies to help you identify the best ways for *you* to learn information in order to help you study for the certification examination.

As an adult learner who has engaged in a comprehensive program of study to prepare for a career in occupational therapy, you will recognize that these are some of the ways you have most likely approached your learning:

- Taken a self-directed approach
- Drawn upon a reservoir of life experiences that serve as a resource for your studying
- Driven by a need to know, do, or find out something new
- Utilized problem-centered, or creative problem-solving strategies to trigger learning experiences
- Been intrinsically motivated to learn as a way to reaching your goal to become an occupational therapy practitioner

It is not unusual however, particularly during transition stages (like preparing to take the certification examination!), for learners to question and re-evaluate their motivation for learning. If you take an adult learning approach to these questions and re-evaluations, it will help you to tap into previous strategies for effective learning, and hopefully assist you with renewing your motivation for study.

The following is a list of helpful strategies that reflect adult learning principles:

1. *Take an active role in planning your studying by setting realistic study goals and expected time commitments.*

2. *Evaluate your progress.* Check off your study goals regularly, demonstrate your knowledge, continually question, and reward yourself for a job well done.

3. *Be open to new experiences – people, resources, materials, and environments.* Think outside of the box, who or what could help you learn more about what it is like to have this disability?

4. *Recognize the value of past experiences.* Recall experiences from your fieldwork, group discussions, and creative projects. Make connections between these and new learning opportunities.

5. *Develop an awareness of what helps you learn best.* Exploit these methods. For example, you may recognize that being able to discuss information in a group helps you to assimilate information. From this, you organize a weekly study group that focuses on preparing to take the certification examination.

6. *Don't be afraid to ask for help.* Academic counseling centers, learning centers, writing centers, reading and/or study skills centers, and student service centers, are just a few resources available to students studying in professional academic programs. Adult learning embraces the notion that it is appropriate to ask for guidance to assist with the learning experience.

> *Remember, being an adult learner means taking responsibility for your learning. Set goals, evaluate, monitor, adapt, develop awareness of past and new experiences, and use resources wisely.*

Scheduling Time for Studying

A common student complaint is that there is not enough time to go around. The time pressures involved in being an adult learner pursuing an occupational therapy education is enormous. Not only does the student typically face tightly scheduled classes, he or she is also expected to carry out several hours of preparation for each hour spent in the classroom, along with studying for tests and writing assignments. This, along with fieldwork and other community-based learning activities, soon add up to a full-time occupation. Many students in an entry-level occupational therapy program find that they have additional commitments related to part-time working and family/social responsibilities taking up even more of their time each week.

The way a student uses time, or wastes time, is largely a matter of habit patterns. By the time a student is ready to graduate from an occupational therapy program and start preparing to study for the certification examination, these study habits will be well developed. Inefficient study habits can be changed however, and it is worth reviewing strategies for time scheduling here, reinforcing adult learning principles of taking responsibility for managing time when studying for the certification examination.

1. *Plan enough time for study.* Review the way you have planned your time to prepare for key assignments during your occupational therapy education. Think of occasions when you achieved a particularly successful grade or outcome, assess the factors that contributed to this including the amount of time you dedicated for preparation. In terms of the preparation you covered, knowledge that was being tested, and type of test/assignment given, estimate in hours/days how much preparation you carried out for this test. Now compare this to the certification examination. What are the similarities and differences between the two tests/assignments? Begin to formulate how much time you will need to optimally study for the certification examination. You are your own best estimator, you know how you work, and how much time you will need to prepare and plan for a successful study schedule. Be honest and realistic with your estimation.

2. *Study at the same time each day.* To develop effective study habits, or modify inefficient study routines, it is recommended that students schedule certain hours that are used for studying throughout the day, every day. This enables a habitual, systematic, study routine to develop and helps to maintain an active approach to learning and preparing for the test.

3. *Make use of free time.* There are many opportunities throughout the day when students could take advantage of additional study time. Carry around a small notebook with the lists, summary statements, and flowcharts you have developed from your studying of specific occupational therapy practice. Use time between classes, riding the bus, waiting for appointments, walking on the treadmill to review your notes. Tap into your critical thinking, question your notes, jot down alternative explanations.

4. *Schedule relaxation time.* Just as your occupational therapy training has emphasized the need for occupational balance, students should build relaxation time into their study schedule. It is more efficient to study hard for a definite period of time, and then stop for a few minutes, than attempt to study on indefinitely. Plan for a 10-15 minute break after every 60-90 minutes of focused study. During this break time, ensure that you move away from your study materials, stretch, and use your other senses such as listening to music or drinking a glass of water, to give your mind a rest from the focused studying. Be disciplined however, to return to your study materials after each allocated break period.

5. *Review regularly.* On a weekly basis, review the progress you have made towards reaching your study goals. Are you still on schedule? Do you need to build in additional study time? Is there flexibility in your schedule to allow for unforeseen events? This review time should prompt you to acknowledge just how well you are doing and build your confidence in preparing to take the certification examination.

6. *Build in time for longer periods of occupational balance.* As well as taking short breaks between periods of focused study, plan for longer periods of "away time" when you can engage in enjoyable activities. Use these scheduled activities as a reward for reaching your study goals and as a way of nurturing your body before returning to your set study schedule.

> *Remember, as an adult learner, you can take responsibility for developing an effective study schedule, build in relaxation time, and be realistic with your time goals.*

Controlling the Study Environment

As an adult learner, you not only need to take responsibility for scheduling time for studying, you need to take control of your study environment. Your occupational therapy training has emphasized the importance of considering the environment in which your clients perform their daily occupations. You can apply the same skill to meet your own needs when designing a study environment to enhance your preparations for taking the certification examination. The following is a list of such environmental strategies:

1. *Set aside a fixed place for study.* This ensures that over time, this place becomes associated with studying behavior, and it will be easier for you to engage in study activities.

2. *Identify factors that increase your ability to focus.* For some people this means making the room as quiet as possible, for others this means putting on some background music. Check if the room is a comfortable temperature, that you have sufficient drinks/snacks close at hand, that your phone is turned off, and that you have all the materials you will need for studying.

3. *Post the goal or goals associated for your planned study session next to your work desk.* This will help you to focus and be an effective motivational tool.

4. *Use symbols, or rituals, to get you in the studying frame of mind.* This might include wearing a particular article of clothing or jewelry, reading a special poem, looking at a favorite picture, or organizing your workspace. Whatever the action, the symbol/ritual will, over time, become associated with studying behavior.

5. *If your mind starts to wander, stand up and look away from your study materials.* Re-connect with the symbol/ritual you used at the start of your study session. Return refreshed and ready to re-focus.

6. *Build in regular review periods.* Post times above your desk when you plan to stop and verbalize what it is you have been studying.

7. *Keep a reminder pad beside you while you study.* Use the pad to jot down thoughts if your mind begins to wander onto other activities besides your studying. Once you have written down the thought, return to your studying. This action will help you to re-focus, while at the same time, provide a reminder to you later of things you have to do.

> *Remember, as an adult learner, you can take control of your study environment. Identify factors that will enhance your study environment and put them into play.*

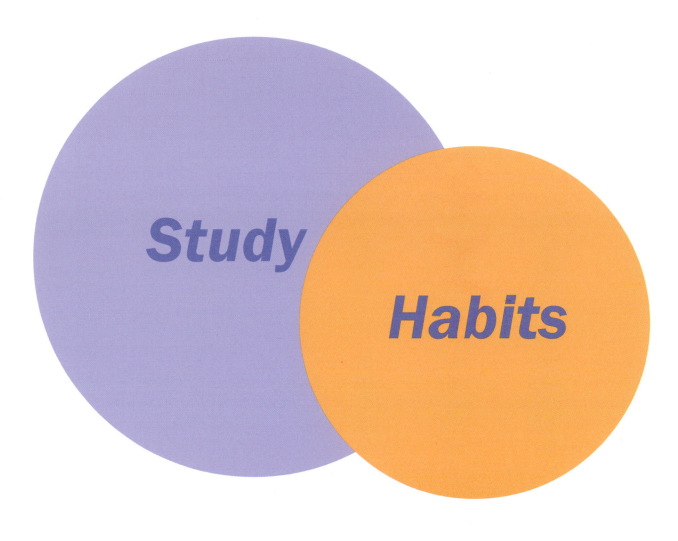

$\mathcal{S}^{\mathit{ection}}$ I of this guide considered adult learning and encouraged the reader to use adult learning principles, such as critical thinking, as a way to organize and conduct studying for the certification examination. This, along with specific emphasis on taking responsibility for managing time and the study environment, provides a strong foundation on which to develop effective study habits. This next section gives an overview of specific study habits. While it is not intended to be an exhaustive list, the reader is encouraged to use the list as a trigger for examining their current study habits, and as a springboard for considering alternative study methods.

Effective Habits for Studying

(Adapted from Covey, S. R. (1989). *The 7 Habits of Highly Effective People.* New York: Simon & Schuster.)

- *Take responsibility for yourself.* Tapping into the principles outlined in the section on adult learning, remind yourself that in order to succeed, you need to make decisions about your priorities (What interventions do you need to study this week?), your time (How much time should I spend reviewing my knowledge on spinal cord levels?), and your resources (I need to coordinate my notes on major mood disorders with the case notes I gathered from my mental health fieldwork).

- *Center yourself around your needs.* Remind yourself, "What is important to me now?" The certification examination can be viewed as the ending of one journey (your academic preparation), and the gateway to your next journey (the start of your professional occupational therapy career). It should be a natural step in your progression towards your chosen career. Use these thoughts to motivate as you set up your study schedule.

- *Follow up on priorities.* Keep to your schedule as far as possible. If you have fallen behind, take steps to review your progress, highlight the reasons for falling behind (Did you set unrealistic study goals? Did you allow others to interrupt your studying?), and try and build in methods to overcome these difficulties in the future (review goals, revise to ensure they are manageable, tell others that you need some undisturbed study time).

- *Congratulate yourself regularly.* Remind yourself of the progress you have made to date – the classes, fieldwork, labs, assignments, and tests completed up to this point. Use your study schedule and completed study goals to highlight the progress you are making towards your goal of taking the certification examination.

- *Consider other solutions.* If you are having difficulty understanding readings from textbooks and class notes, think of alternative ways for you to make sense of this material. For example, you might consider talking it through with one of your professors, revisiting a fieldwork site, or joining a peer study group.

> *Remind yourself of the progress you have made to date. Use your study schedule and completed study tasks to highlight the progress you are making towards your goal.*

Concentrating When Studying

Just as we all have the ability to concentrate, there will be times when it is difficult for us to remain focused. Our mind may wander from one topic to another, worries about the consequences of not doing well on the test, allowing outside distractions to interfere with our study routine, and finding the material difficult or uninteresting can contribute to loss of concentration while trying to study. There are two effective methods for increasing ability to concentrate.

1. *Scheduled Worry Time.* Set aside a specific time each day to think about the things that keep entering your mind and interfere with your studying. When you become aware of a distracting thought, remind yourself that you have a special time to think about them. Let the thought go, and keep your appointment to worry or think about those distracting issues at the time you have scheduled for these. Let your mind return to focus on your immediate activity of studying.

2. *Be Here Now.* When you notice your thoughts wandering, say to yourself, "Be here now." Gently bring your attention back to where you want it to be – your notes on developmental milestones, for example. If your mind wanders again, repeat the phrase "Be here now." and gently bring your attention back. Continually practice this technique and you should notice that the period of time between your straying thoughts gets a little longer each time. Be patient and keep at it.

Using Memory Effectively

While acronyms (invented combination of letters), acrostic (invented sentence where first letter of each word is a cue to an idea you need to remember), rhyme-keys, and chaining are recognized techniques for recalling systems or lists of information (and they are described at length in many other generic study guide texts), they are perhaps not the most effective methods for studying and recalling material in preparation for NBCOT's certification examination. Test items on this examination rely on candidates demonstrating their knowledge as it applies to the practice of occupational therapy.

Alternative methods should include using memory of situations and experiences as applied to practice. For example, when studying the ulnar nerve, the candidate may associate actions of the flexor muscles with specific tasks such as holding a pencil or utensil. Fieldwork experiences may also act as a strong memory aid where candidates recall working with a particular individual who had a similar disability to the ones presented on the examination.

Using memory in this sense will enable you to apply your knowledge to the practice of occupational therapy.

Thinking Aloud

Through your learning about human development during your occupational therapy education, you are probably familiar with the term "private speech." Private speech is an accepted way for infants and children to think aloud or say what they are thinking as a way of demonstrating knowledge. Children use private speech to practice words, express ideas, form sentences, and as a way to make sense of their external world. Thinking aloud is essential to early learning. As we grow older, thinking aloud or private speech, becomes internalized. However, whenever we encounter unfamiliar or demanding activities in our adult lives, we can use private speech as a way to overcome obstacles and acquire new skills.

The more we engage our brain on multiple levels, the more we are able to make connections and retain what we learn. We can apply these same techniques to our study habits. As well as reading, we can create images, listen, talk with others, and talk with ourselves about the concepts we are learning. Some of us like to talk things through with someone else as a way of increasing our understanding, and others do not need another person around to talk with in this process. Using multiple senses and experiences to process and reinforce our learning is an individualized process, but one that can be very effective in helping to understand and retain knowledge.

> **Remember to engage your brain on multiple levels while studying. Utilize various techniques, senses and experiences to process and reinforce your learning.**

Avoiding Procrastination

Procrastination can stop you from achieving the study goals you wish to reach. Here are some ways to help overcome procrastination:

Ask yourself, "What is it that I want to do?"

- What is your final objective, the end result?
  I want to review my notes on occupational therapy frames of reference.

- What are the major steps to get there?
  I need to locate my class notes.
  I need to check out the theory book from the library.
  I need to access my fieldwork journal where I wrote a case study using 3 major frames of reference.
  I need to prepare a grid showing the major frames of reference for my study group.

- What have you done so far?
  I've got the book from the library.
  I've found my fieldwork journal.
  I've bought some large sheets of grid paper and marker pens.

Next ask yourself, "Why do I want to do this?"

- What is your biggest motivation?
  I want to have all the frames of reference clear in my mind.
  I'd like to apply theoretical concepts to practice application.
  I need to feel I am contributing to the study group.
  I want to feel prepared for the certification exam.

- What other positive results will flow from achieving this goal?
  I can talk about my knowledge during recruitment interviews.
  I can use them to aid my documentation when writing up treatment plans in the future.
  I can assist members in my study group to understand the similarities and differences between the theories.

List what stands in your way:

- What is in your power to change?

    If I chose to review a frame of reference that I'm interested in first, it will help me to feel motivated to study the others.

    I don't want to prepare this grid in case I mess it up, but if I draft it on the computer I can build it up gradually.

    There are so many to cover, I'll never get through them all. If I group them together into categories, they will be more manageable for me to study.

- What resources beside yourself do you need?

    I could use some help with drawing up this grid. I am going to ask one other member from the study group to work on this with me.

- What will happen if I don't progress?

    I won't know this material.

    There will be questions on the examination that I can't answer.

    I will let my study group down.

- Develop your plan by:

    Setting realistic goals for yourself.

    Defining how much time each goal will take to realize.

    Building in rewards.

    Building in time for review.

    Fantasizing – see yourself succeeding!

- Admit to mistakes:

    Everyone makes them, it is part of the learning experience.

    Distractions - build extra time into your study schedule, and try to re-focus on the task.

    Emotion – we all get frustrated at times, especially when things are not going as well as we had planned. Turn that frustration around, and acknowledge that you are doing something about it.

Index Study Systems

Using index study systems is an effective strategy to evaluate how well you know and understand the material you have studied. Follow these steps to build up your own index study system:

- As you read through your study notes, write down potential test questions about the material on one side of an index card:

    How does macular degeneration affect the person's ability to do grooming activities?

    What recommendations could the occupational therapy practitioner make to a homemaker with macular degeneration?

- On the other side of the card, write an explanation in answer to your question posted. Include any references or texts you have used during your studying to validate your response.

    A person with macular degeneration will have difficulty distinguishing visual details such as variations in colors, patterns and contrast. Activities such as medication management, putting on make-up, or choosing clothing may be difficult for the individual to complete. (Reference: Early, M.B. (2006). Physical Dysfunction Practice Skills for the Occupational Therapy Assistant (2nd Ed.). St Louis: Elsevier Mosby (pages 443-4).

- When you have completed writing up a series of index cards about a particular subject, shuffle the cards. Look at the card on top and read the question. Try to answer it in your own words. If you experience difficulty, turn the card over and review the answer you have written.

- Keep going through the deck until you know all the information you have catalogued.

- Carry the cards with you – take advantage of free time to review your knowledge.

- Use the cards to study with your peer group. Test each other, check that others understand your explanations, come up with alternative solutions to the problems posted.

Cooperative and Collaborative Learning

Your occupational therapy education has provided many opportunities for you to experience cooperative and collaborative learning opportunities. This is an interactive learning approach where group members develop and share a common goal, contribute understanding of specific problems, post questions, offer insights and solutions. Many students find it effective to use a similar approach for studying to take the certification examination.

What makes an effective study group?

- Use understanding of group process principles.
- Keep the group to a manageable size (maximum of six).
- Assign a group leader.
- Choose members who will bring specific strengths to the group.
- Empower members to contribute.
- Encourage commitment.
- Share group operating principles and responsibilities such as:
  - Commitment to attend, preparation, and starting meetings on time.
  - Having discussions and disagreements that focus on issues, not personal criticism.
  - Taking responsibility to share tasks and carry them out on time.

Process of setting up a study group:

- Set goals, define how often and with what means you will communicate, evaluate progress, make decisions, and resolve conflict.
- Define resources, especially someone who can provide direction, supervision, counsel, and even arbitrate.
- Schedule review of your progress and communication to discuss what is working, and what is not working.

Test-Taking Strategies

*S*ection II presented an array of strategies to encourage effective study habits. This next section examines general test-taking strategies including what to do before, during, and after the test, tips for overcoming test anxiety, and guidelines for answering multiple-choice items.

Before, During, and After the Test

Before the test:

Remind yourself of the progress you have made to date. You have already completed an occupational therapy program. You have taken many academic courses, successfully completed assignments, and passed several major tests. Think back to how much you knew about occupational therapy at the start of your program, compared to how much you know now. View the certification examination as just one step further towards your goal of becoming an occupational therapy practitioner. You have taken many steps up to this point, and this is one of the last steps you will need to take towards your career goal.

Continue to set realistic study goals, identifying your strengths and addressing any weaknesses in your knowledge. Use the Examination Readiness Tool in Appendix A to help you. Regularly review your progress, check off your study goals, seek additional help for information you are finding difficult to understand, build in regular breaks, and try and predict how the information you are studying might be presented on the test. Remember that items on the certification examination are always practice-based. Regularly demonstrate the knowledge you have acquired through: revising your study notes, using index systems, contributing to a study group, using lists, charts, and writing review papers.

The night before the test:

- Do not engage in last minute cramming. If you have followed a well-planned study schedule, there is no need for you to do last minute cramming.
- Make sure you know the exact site of the examination center. Estimate how long it will take you to get there and build in extra time for traffic, taking the wrong turn, unforeseen circumstances. Make sure your vehicle has gas, and is in full working order.
- Make sure you have all the documentation you will need to take with you to the test site – refer to the latest copy of the NBCOT Candidate Handbook online at *www.nbcot.org*.
- Pack earplugs to bring along to test site if you feel this will help your concentration as you take the examination.
- Engage in some form of physical activity. This will help to alleviate pretest nerves.
- Decide what clothes you plan to wear – comfort and layered clothing are the key considerations. Try to get a good night's sleep, and remember to set the alarm clock.

The day of the test:

- Arrive at the test site early.
- Try not to talk to others taking the same test – anxiety can be contagious.
- Take some deep, slow breaths.
- Remind yourself how well you have done up to this point.
- Organize your workspace – familiarize yourself with the computer and ensure you can see a watch/ clock.
- Ask for headphones or use your earplugs if you know you will be distracted by others working around you.

- Ensure your seat feels comfortable, and sit in an upright position.
- Advise the test center proctor of any problems or concerns you have regarding the test environment prior to beginning the test.

During the test:

- Take the tutorial. Time for completing the tutorial is not deducted from your actual exam time.
- Read all instructions VERY CAREFULLY before starting to answer the test questions.
- Divide up the time given for the test. There will be 200 test items on the COTA certification examination. Divide the time you have been given (4 hours unless you have been granted a special accommodation) by 200, and build in time so you can review the entire test prior to finishing. Use markers after each hour so you can keep yourself on schedule.
- Pace your energy levels. Answer questions you are relatively sure about first, this will speed up your progress allowing you to spend more time on those you are less certain about.
- Use erasable board and marker pen (this will be provided at the test site) to help you organize and clarify your thinking.
- Change your position regularly – stretch, drop your shoulders, open and close your fingers, shift in your chair.
- Flag questions you are uncertain about, you will be able to return to these later as time permits.
- Don't panic if other people in the exam room finish before you do. You do not need to leave the test room until you have used all of the allotted time; or reviewed all items and ensured that you have answered each question.
- Only change an answer you have given if you are really sure about it. The answer that comes to mind first is often correct. Reviewing with an anxious mind and changing answers when you are not certain can do more harm than good.
- Rely on your knowledge and do not watch for patterns. Noticing that the last four answers are always the third choice is not a good reason to change your answer. The test answers are randomized.
- If you experience problems during the exam, inform the test center proctor.

After the test:

- Resist the urge to talk through test items and potential answers with your peer group. You have completed the exam, and it is too late to change your answers now.
- Resist the urge to open up your study notes, texts, and review guides for the same reason given above.
- Remember, it is against NBCOT's Candidate/Certificant Code of Conduct to discuss test items with other candidates, or to record test information from memory.
- Relax. You have waited for this moment for a long time, you can do no more, reward yourself for completing this stage.
- If you do wish to post an exam challenge, ensure you do this in writing, and within the timelines given in the NBCOT *Certification Examination Handbook,* and on page 26 of this guide.

Overcoming Test Anxiety

It is of course, very natural to experience a level of anxiety prior to sitting for the certification examination. This is a day that you have been working towards for a long period of time, and marks your passage towards achieving your career goal. Your occupational therapy education has provided you with many instances when anxiety has been a natural response—interviewing your first real patient, arriving at your first day of fieldwork, giving a formal presentation in front of a large audience. Remind yourself that a certain amount of anxiety can actually be very beneficial to your performance. It heightens your awareness and enables you to remain alert. Anxiety can become a problem however, if it lasts too long and starts to interfere with your ability to concentrate.

The following are some tips to help you manage your anxiety:

- Prepare, prepare, prepare. This includes following a realistic and well planned study schedule, as well as preparing physically for getting to the test site on time.
- Ensure you have exercised, eaten, and had a good night's sleep.
- Use cue cards to remind you how well you have done.
- View the test as an opportunity to demonstrate how much you know and have achieved.
- Remember, the examination is not designed to trick you.
- Engage in relaxation techniques – visualization, controlled breathing, tensing and relaxing muscles groups.
- Change position, visit the restroom, have a drink of water.

If you notice that at times you have not been able to manage your anxiety levels, and that this has interfered with your ability to perform on exams, seek help from a qualified professional. Your student counseling center, or healthcare provider will be able to recommend help available to you.

Guidelines for Answering Multiple-Choice Questions

NBCOT uses multiple-choice test items for the COTA certification examination. The format for the multiple-choice test items is as follows:

- Each item has a stem or premise. This is usually in the form of a written statement, or series of statements. Stems always relate to the knowledge, skills, and abilities relevant to actual practice at the entry-level. The following is an example of a stem:

  A homemaker who has multiple sclerosis wants to continue to be independent with self-care tasks including cooking meals and doing laundry. Which interventions should the COTA use INITIALLY to promote progress toward this goal?

- Following the stem, there are four possible answers posted. There is only ONE correct answer to the stem/premise, the other three options are distractors. It may be that all the answers provided are plausible to some degree, but there is only one choice that is the **BEST** response. Candidates need to solicit the best response based on all the information presented in the stem. The following are the four possible answers posted for the example above:

  A. *Teach work simplification, pacing and energy conservation techniques.*
  B. *Collaborate with the client to discuss expectations and prioritize needs.*
  C. *Recommend environmental modifications that will improve performance.*
  D. *Talk with the family about the impact of the disease on role performance.*

- Read the whole question carefully. Note key words. In the above question, the key words are: initially; homemaker; multiple sclerosis; independent; self-care tasks; and interventions.

- Ask yourself, "What is this question really asking?" In the above question, it is asking about your knowledge of initially prioritizing interventions in order to meet client-centered goals for a homemaker who has multiple sclerosis.

- Eliminate response options you know are wrong. In the above example, response option D is clearly incorrect – there is no information in the stem to suggest this person has family involvement. Options A and C are plausible – and certainly may be things you could include in an intervention. However, remember the question is asking about your knowledge of initially meeting client-centered goals. Therefore response option B is the correct answer. This response takes into account the need to collaborate with the client and prioritize their needs before commencing intervention activities.

- Although there is never more than one correct answer, candidates may think there are several possibilities posted, and find it difficult to choose between the options. If this is the case, re-read the stem. Key words in the stem that state, "The **FIRST** thing the COTA should do is," "The **BEST** thing the COTA should do," or "The **INITIAL** response by the COTA should be," will provide the clues needed to determine the correct response.

- Practice answering the sample multiple-choice questions in Section V of this study guide. Remember, read and re-read the stem. Ask yourself, "What is this question really asking?" Eliminate obvious incorrect answers. Re-read the information provided in the stem for clues needed to determine the correct response. Make your decision about the answer based on information provided in the stem.

- Although it can be very useful, when considering test items, to remember similar patients you have worked with during your fieldwork, there may be a danger that you dismiss key information provided in the item stem. Remember, the correct answer only applies to the scenario posted in the stem, which may not exactly match circumstances under which you have worked with patients during fieldwork. All your decisions should; therefore, be based on the facts presented in the stem statements.

- Refer to Appendix C for a list of abbreviations that are used on the certification examination. Appendix D provides a list of the interventions, service components, and settings commonly used on the certification examination.

> *Remember, taking the certification examination brings you one step further toward your goal of becoming an occupational therapy practitioner. Remind yourself of the progress you have made to get to this point!*

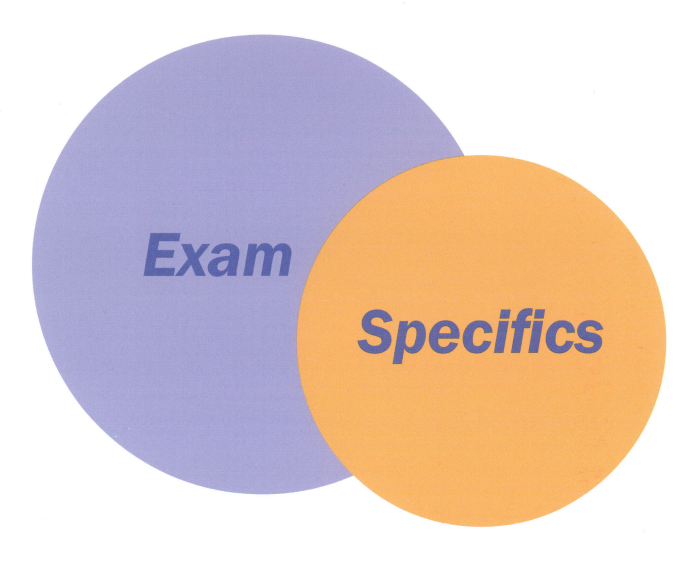

Exam

Specifics

Background

Following certification industry standards, NBCOT certification examinations are constructed based on the results of practice analysis studies. The ultimate goal of practice analysis studies are to ensure that there is a representative linkage of test content to practice, making certain that the credentialing examination contains meaningful indicators of competence, and providing evidence that supports the examination's content validity of current occupational therapy practice. The periodic performance of practice analysis studies assists NBCOT with evaluating the validity of the test specifications that guide content distribution of the credentialing examinations. Because the practice of occupational therapy changes and evolves over time, practice analysis studies are conducted by NBCOT on a regular basis.

NBCOT conducted a practice analysis study of certified occupational therapy assistant practice in 2007. The results from this study were used to construct examination test blueprints for administrations starting January 2009.

Building upon previous studies, a large-scale survey was used with entry level COTA practitioners who were asked to evaluate job requirements on criticality and frequency rating scales. The job requirements were classified as the domains, tasks, knowledge and skills required for current occupational therapy assistant practice.

- **Domains** broadly define the major performance components of the profession.
- **Tasks** describe activities that are performed in each domain (i.e., things that practitioners do).
- **Knowledge** statements describe the information required to perform each task competently.
- **Skills** describe the abilities needed by the Certificant to implement the task. Samples of domain, task, knowledge and skill statements are as follows:

Domain:	Select and implement evidence-based interventions to support participation in areas of occupation throughout the continuum of care
Task:	Modify intervention methods and techniques based on the client's needs and responses in order to promote occupational performance
Knowledge of:	Methods of adapting the intervention environment based on medical status and behavioral responses to maximize participation in areas of occupation
Skill:	Adapting the environment to support participation during the intervention

The results of the survey were analyzed to identify the most critical and frequently performed tasks by the COTA survey respondents. Weights were then established to determine the relative proportion of test items devoted to each of the three domain areas established for the COTA examination blueprints. Table 4.1 displays the COTA blueprint specifications derived from the results of the 2007 NBCOT practice analysis study. These blueprints will guide examination development for the NBCOT COTA certification examinations beginning January 2009.

The percentage of items in each domain area shown on page 23 remains constant on each exam form of the COTA certification examination. There are multiple task, knowledge, and skill statements for each of the three domain areas. For a full overview of task, knowledge, and skill statements specific to each of the three domain areas for the COTA certification examination, please see Appendix E.

Table 4.1. COTA Blueprint Specifications Based on the 2007 Practice Analysis Study –
Implementation January 2009 examination administrations

Domain	Description	Percent of Exam
01	Gather information and formulate conclusions regarding the client's needs and priorities to develop a client-centered intervention plan	33%
02	Select and implement evidence-based interventions to support participation in areas of occupation throughout the continuum of care	47%
03	Uphold professional standards and responsibilities to promote quality in practice	20%

Exam Construction

NBCOT contracts with a professional testing agency who is responsible for meeting test specifications including item construction and ensuring that accepted psychometric principles in test construction are met. The testing agency assists NBCOT during test development by assuring the content validity, reliability and security of the NBCOT examinations.

Each item (question) appearing on the COTA examination has been developed to assess essential knowledge acceptable for entry-level performance by an occupational therapy assistant. In addition, the items are designed to differentiate from an individual whose knowledge is acceptable for certification and an individual whose knowledge is not acceptable for certification. All items have been subjected to multiple rigorous reviews. Examination items are carefully reviewed for bias, making sure that the context, setting, language, descriptions, terminology, and content of the items are free of stereotype and equally appropriate for all segments of the candidate population.

The COTA examination consists of 200 multiple-choice items. Of these 200 items, a number are scored and a number are unscored items. The unscored items are intermingled with the scored items and are indistinguishable to the testing candidate. A scored exam item is an item that is considered in the pass/fail status of a candidate. Each examination item is psychometrically analyzed prior to use on the examination as a scored item. As a matter of practice, examination items are pre-tested; however, pre-test items are not included in a candidate's examination score. After pre-test items have a fixed number of examination exposures, the items are psychometrically analyzed to determine if they satisfy credentialing standards for valid and reliable test questions. If the items satisfy these standards, they are included in the item bank for future use.

In summary, no scoreable item is included on the certification examination that does not 1) satisfy the examination blueprint specifications resulting from the practice analysis study, 2) meet development standards described above, or 3) satisfy the psychometric standards for a scoreable exam item.

Standard Setting, Equating, & Scoring

All NBCOT certification examinations are criterion referenced. This means in order to pass the examination, the candidate must obtain a score equal to – or higher than – the minimum passing score. The minimum passing score represents an absolute standard and does not depend on the performance of other candidates taking the same examination. The minimum passing score on the COTA certification examination is set by content experts using widely recognized standard setting methodologies.

NBCOT develops multiple forms of their certification examinations to ensure security and integrity of the examination. Every form employs a unique combination of test items so that no two forms are identical but all forms are equal in difficulty level.

NBCOT uses a scaled scoring procedure to determine a candidate's final score. The scaled score is not a "number correct" or "percent correct" score. Raw scores are converted to scaled scores that represent equivalent levels of achievement regardless of test form. The passing point for NBCOT's COTA certification examination is set at 450 points, with the lowest possible score set at 300 and the highest possible score set at 600 points. Candidates must obtain a scaled score of at least 450 points in order to pass the examination. For more information on the psychometric principles that form the foundations of the NBCOT certification examinations, please refer to *www.nbcot.org*.

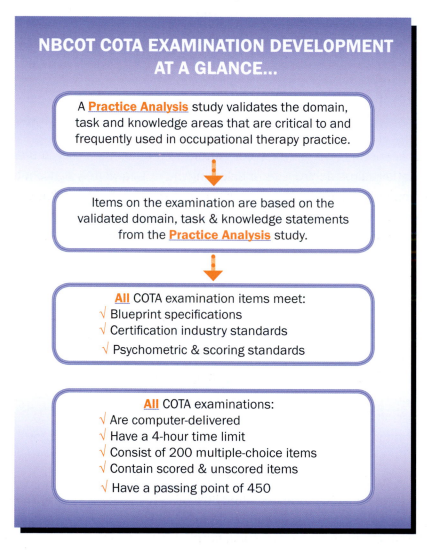

NBCOT COTA EXAMINATION DEVELOPMENT AT A GLANCE...

A **Practice Analysis** study validates the domain, task and knowledge areas that are critical to and frequently used in occupational therapy practice.

Items on the examination are based on the validated domain, task & knowledge statements from the **Practice Analysis** study.

All COTA examination items meet:
√ Blueprint specifications
√ Certification industry standards
√ Psychometric & scoring standards

All COTA examinations:
√ Are computer-delivered
√ Have a 4-hour time limit
√ Consist of 200 multiple-choice items
√ Contain scored & unscored items
√ Have a passing point of 450

Examination Preparation Tools

In addition to this study guide, NBCOT has developed a number of resources to assist examination candidates with their test preparation; for example, the COTA Examination Readiness Tool (see Appendix A) and online COTA practice tests. All official NBCOT study tools are developed to meet the current examination blueprint specifications with items that have been developed in the same manner as those used on the actual certification examination. For details of the official NBCOT study tools, visit *www.nbcot.org*.

TEST ADMINISTRATION

Taking Computer-Based Tests

Test centers are built to standard specifications and vary primarily on the basis of size. NBCOT candidates arriving at the test site must have a valid, current, government-issued ID, and must sign the roster. Private modular workstations provide ample workspace, comfortable seating, and lighting. Proctors monitor the testing process through an observation window and from within the testing room. Parabolic mirrors mounted on the walls assist proctors in observing the testing process. All testing sessions are videotaped and audio-monitored. During the testing session, people taking examinations other than the NBCOT examinations may be in the testing room.

The test is administered at a standard work station. The regular computer table/desks are about 28" from the floor. All of the chairs are adjustable in height from at least 15 1/2" from the floor to 20 1/2." Some chairs have even more range than that. Chairs do have armrests. Every site has 2-foot stools available to candidates should feet not reach the floor with chair adjustment. The monitors can be pointed upward or downward, or turned from one side to another. Should the initial monitor placement result in glare, an adjustment such as this will resolve that issue.

Computer knowledge is not required to take a computerized examination. Before the examination begins, an introductory tutorial explains the process of selecting answers and moving from question to question. The time candidates spend on the tutorial does NOT count against the time allotted for the examination. Most candidates take approximately five to 10 minutes to complete the tutorial. Candidates are strongly encouraged to use the tutorial prior to taking the examination, and may select their answers using either the keyboard or the mouse. COTA examination candidates are allotted four (4) hours to complete the examination.

The test questions are presented one at a time on the monitor. The standard font size is 12 points. There is a bar at the bottom of the screen that enables moving to a final summary page, and to other questions. Candidates can skip forward or backward through the examination, and review questions at any point during their testing session. Candidates may review and change answers at any time prior to FINAL submission. The testing software contains a feature that allows candidates to mark questions that they might wish to review later, if time permits. The test site will provide an erasable board and marker pen. These must be turned in when the exam is over. Candidates may not bring their own scratch paper or pencil/pen.

All test situations are subject to some noise and distraction. In a computer-based setting, other test-takers may be taking essay exams, so there may be some keyboarding sounds from test-takers nearby. The test center staff may also be providing some brief assistance to other test-takers in the room. If a candidate is concerned that these situations may be distracting, earplugs are permitted. Candidates are allowed to use earplugs that are supplied by the testing center, or they may bring their own. Earplugs are not automatically distributed to candidates. Candidates must ask test center staff for them. However, because there is no guarantee of the availability of earplugs, candidates who believe that they will need earplugs are strongly advised to bring their own. Note that only small "in-the-ear" earplugs are allowed. Large "room silencers" or any headphone-types of equipment are not allowed without prior special accommodations approval.

Candidates may stop and take a break, go to the restroom, or get some water or a snack from a locker. Breaks may be taken at any time, and as often as is reasonable and necessary. The exam time continues to run during any breaks. For more details on test administration, refer to the current copy of the NBCOT *Certification Examination Handbook*.

Accommodations

In compliance with the Americans with Disabilities Act (ADA), NBCOT makes special testing arrangements for candidates with professionally diagnosed and documented disabilities. Under the ADA, a disability is defined as "a physical or mental impairment that substantially limits one or more major life activities" (e.g., caring for one's self, performing manual tasks, walking, seeing, breathing, learning, working). If you intend to apply for special testing accommodations in order to take the COTA certification examination, you need to provide comprehensive documentation supporting your diagnosis, and the impact of the disability on major life activity. Submit the documentation AFTER you have filed your examination application. A review is then conducted per ADA guidelines. An Authorization to Test (ATT) letter will be sent only after the decision about the special accommodations request is final. Please refer to information about Special Accommodations online at *www.nbcot.org*.

Unfortunate Events

Examination Content Challenges, Administration Complaints, and Appeals

A candidate may challenge the content of specific test items (include as much specific information as possible about the test item) or file a complaint regarding the administration of the examination by sending a letter describing the basis for the content challenge or administrative complaint and including pertinent information. The letter of challenge or complaint must be POSTMARKED NO LATER THAN 24 HOURS AFTER THE CANDIDATE TAKES THE EXAMINATION AND SENT VIA TRACEABLE MAIL/DELIVERY – SIGNATURE OF RECEIPT REQUIRED (e.g., certified mail) to NBCOT.

With regard to a letter of administrative complaint or content challenge, NBCOT will investigate and respond in writing to the candidate. A candidate may appeal the decision by sending a letter describing the justification of the appeal. This letter of appeal must be received by NBCOT no later than 21 days after the candidate's receipt of the notification of NBCOT's decision. Please refer to the latest NBCOT *Certification Examination Handbook* online at *www.nbcot.org*.

Failing the Examination

Unfortunately, not every candidate who takes NBCOT's certification examinations will achieve a successful passing score. While it is obviously very disappointing to receive notification that you did not meet the passing requirement (a scaled score of 450 points or above), it is essential to address the consequences of this occurrence. A candidate's test score (including a failing score) will only be reported to the candidate, and to a state licensing board, if the candidate requested for their score transfer reports to be sent to a state regulatory board(s). Without the candidate's written permission, no other persons will be informed of the candidate's failed score. Not passing the NBCOT certification examination may impact the candidate's plans to commence an occupational therapy job position. It is the candidate's responsibility to inform any potential employer that they are not currently certified, if they did not successfully pass the NBCOT certification examination and are seeking employment as a COTA. Candidates need to contact state regulatory entities for specific information regarding temporary licenses.

Candidates who fail the certification examination will be informed as to when they are able to schedule a subsequent examination within a specific examination eligibility period. The eligibility period can begin no sooner than 45 days from the test date shown on the candidate's score report. A new ATT letter will be sent to the candidate and this will specify the next examination eligibility period based on the 45-day end-date and receipt of the new application.

Preparing to Re-Take the Certification Examination
There may be many reasons for a candidate failing NBCOT's certification examination. Reflecting on potential reasons is an important first step in preparing to re-take the examination. These reasons may include:

- Poor test-taking strategies
- Inadequate study habits
- Lack of preparation
- Test anxiety
- External stresses

After identifying potential reasons, revisit the initial sections in this study guide to help develop a plan of action. Pay particular attention to the sections on Adult Learning, Developing Effective Study Habits, and General Test-Taking Strategies. Use the sample multiple-choice items at the end of this study guide to help familiarize yourself with the format and domain areas of the certification examination. For any incorrect responses, use the rationales and follow-up references to help guide your study and preparation.

Interpreting The Score Reports
Candidates who fail the NBCOT COTA certification examination will be provided with a score report that outlines the candidate's scaled score for each of the domain areas represented in the certification examination. In addition, information regarding the average U.S. new graduate candidate's scaled scores across domains is also included.

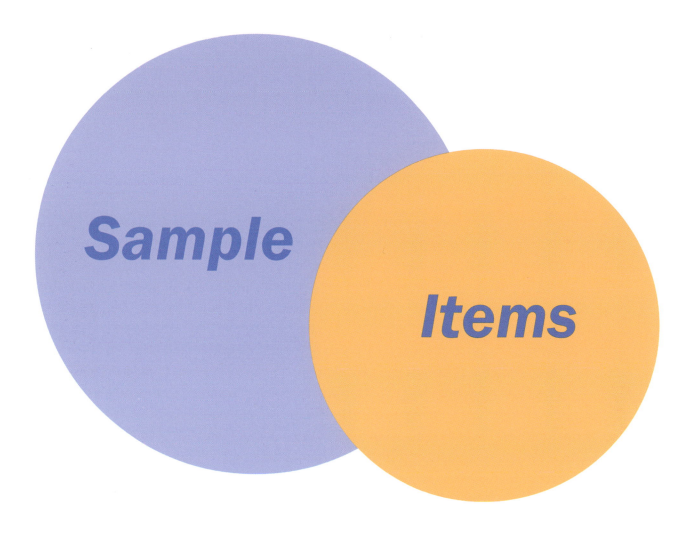

Sample Items

The 2007 Blueprint Specifications for the COTA validated domain, task, and knowledge statements (see Appendix E) provides the basis for the COTA certification examination item development. The outline for the examination is based upon the three domain areas identified in the blueprint, and the percentage for each domain weight (the approximate percent of items from the domain appearing on each examination) is listed on page 23.

This section consists of 100 COTA multiple-choice sample items across all three domain areas. Examples of domain-specific test items are grouped together under each domain heading for learning purposes in this study guide. However, candidates should take note that the items on the actual certification examination will appear in random order.

It is recommended that candidates use these sample items in the following ways:

- Start by completing the Examination Readiness Tool in Appendix A. This will highlight areas of strength and weakness.
- Next, read and answer the sample items. As a guide to develop an effective study plan, identify items that you score incorrectly. Read the rationale for the correct response, and follow up by studying the reference materials listed.
- Practice taking a timed test. There are 100 multiple-choice items included in this section. The actual certification examination will consist of 200 questions. If you have not been granted a special accommodation, you will be allocated four hours in which to complete the test. Therefore, practice answering the items in this section within a two-hour period.
- Use the 2007 Blueprint Specifications (Appendix E) to identify specific domain areas with subsequent task and knowledge statements to enhance your studying and preparation efforts.
- After answering the sample items, compare your answers to the answer key on page 56.
- For incorrect answers, refer to the answer section beginning on page 57. Read the rationale for the correct answer and explanations for the incorrect answers. Use the references provided for additional information to enhance your studying.
- Use this experience to guide discussion in your study groups or further guide individual examination preparation efforts.

The following multiple-choice items are samples related to Domain Area 1:

Gather information and formulate conclusions regarding the client's needs and priorities to develop a client-centered intervention plan

1. A supervising OTR asks a newly certified COTA to perform a standardized manual muscle test on a client. The COTA has only administered this test on classmates when in school; and received an excellent score on the final laboratory exam. Which action should the COTA take **INITIALLY** in response to this request?

    1. Plan to administer the assessment after reviewing class notes.
    2. Ask the OTR for clarification as to which muscles are supposed to be tested.
    3. Talk with the OTR about establishing service competency for the test.
    4. Arrange for a colleague to observe so inter-rater reliability can be established.

2. What is the **PRIMARY** purpose for administering a standardized occupational performance survey to clients who are participating in an inpatient hand rehabilitation group activity?

    1. To determine if the clients need clarification on some of the rehab techniques
    2. To assess the clients' overall satisfaction with the rehabilitation
    3. To test the clients' memory about the information presented during a session
    4. To collect information about the impact of the injury on the clients' activities

3. A multidisciplinary team of a skilled nursing facility is developing a plan of care for an individual who has mild dementia and has urinary incontinence. What is the **PRIMARY** role of the COTA when coordinating care related to the individual's incontinence issues?

    1. Reporting the impact of the incontinence on social interactions
    2. Recommending environmental and clothing adaptations
    3. Outlining methods to nursing for maintaining a daily bladder record
    4. Identifying support systems to help implement a bladder program

4. Which type of information is the school-based COTA **PRIMARILY** responsible for reporting during a student's IEP review?

    1. Age-appropriate leisure activities that the student should be able to complete
    2. Progress the student has made in school-related activities over the past year
    3. Normative comparisons using perceptual-motor test scores
    4. Receptive and expressive language the student currently uses

5.   What is the **PRIMARY** purpose for writing client-centered goals as part of an intervention plan?

   1.   Informing other healthcare professionals about expected client outcomes
   2.   Reflecting realistic accomplishments that the client wants to achieve
   3.   Outlining tasks that the therapist intends to accomplish with the client
   4.   Maximizing reimbursement for client services from third-party payors

6.   At the beginning of an assertiveness training program, the COTA asks the participants to complete a questionnaire asking about situations in which they believe they are not assertive and want to change. What is the **PRIMARY** purpose for administering this questionnaire?

   1.   Identifying areas of strengths and weaknesses
   2.   Promoting socialization among group members
   3.   Determining issues the group members want to address
   4.   Evaluating the individual's self-assessment skills

7.   Residents at an assisted living facility are asking for more staff assistance during meals in the dining room due to problems associated with low vision. Which recommendation should the COTA make based on this change?

   1.   Interview the residents to identify their individual needs during meals.
   2.   Train staff about how to respond to the residents' questions during meal times.
   3.   Serve food on brightly colored trays with each food group on a separate plate.
   4.   Teach residents who do not have visual deficits how to assist as needed.

8.   Which information is **MOST IMPORTANT** to verify prior to providing a home program to a client who has had a CVA and is participating in outpatient OT?

   1.   The extent to which the client understands the rationale for the program
   2.   The client's ability to follow through with the self-directed program
   3.   The client's capacity to verbalize the home program instructions
   4.   The amount of family support available to the client on a daily basis

9.   An inpatient who has Stage 3 Alzheimer's disease (moderate to moderately severe decline in cognition) has difficulty sequencing steps for self-care activities and is easily frustrated. The patient is preparing for discharge to live in the family home with adult children. Which information should the COTA contribute to this patient's discharge planning process?

   1.   Recommendations for a home health aide to make daily visits to the family home
   2.   Strategies the patient's family can use to cope with the patient's functional decline
   3.   Techniques that can be used at home to ensure the patient independently completes self-care
   4.   Instructions to the family about medication requirements and daily dosage routines

10. An inpatient who is recovering from depression is preparing for discharge from an acute psychiatric facility to live at home alone. The patient recently retired from a religious profession. Which of the following is an effective client-centered approach to use with this patient?

 1. Exploring a variety of potential vocational skills with the patient
 2. Recommending the patient attend a support group after discharge
 3. Encouraging the patient to attend church-sponsored activities
 4. Asking the patient open-ended questions about preferred leisure activities

11. While leading an ADL group in a long-term care facility, a COTA notices that several residents are wearing splints incorrectly. What action should the COTA take in response to this observation?

 1. Instruct the family members about splint application and skin checks.
 2. Review correct splint application with the residents and nursing staff.
 3. Present a staff inservice about consequences of incorrect splint application.
 4. Adjust the splints for a correct fit and follow up frequently.

12. An individual who had a recent TBI has hemiparesis, moderate short-term memory deficits and impulsiveness, and requires cueing for safety during BADL. Discharge plans are for the individual to transition from the inpatient rehabilitation facility to live at home with a caregiver. Which caregiver instruction should be included in the discharge plans to maximize the individual's safety for showering at home?

 1. Be sure the individual holds onto a grab bar when standing to take a shower.
 2. Provide stand-by assistance and have the individual sit on a tub bench.
 3. Encourage the individual to use a long-handle reacher and a bath mitt.
 4. Have the individual step onto a bath towel after getting out of the shower.

13. A client who is in the recovery phase of Guillain-Barré syndrome identifies a long-term goal of being able to lift their four-month-old infant in and out of the crib. The client has met the short-term goal of being able to lift a 10-pound weight from the floor to a table. Which statement is the **BEST** example of a short-term goal to include as part of the next phase of intervention?

 1. "Client will be able to safely lifts 15 pounds from the floor to the table five out of five times without assistance."
 2. "Client will verbalize methods for using proper body mechanics for lifting objects over 50 pounds."
 3. "Client will lift the infant from the floor to their lap from a seated position."
 4. "Client will complete at least three child-care activities prior to being left alone with the infant."

14. A COTA has been working with a 4-year-old child to help the child learn cause-and-effect relationships through the use of a switch-operated toy. The child has progressed from not pressing the switch at all, to inconsistently pressing the switch within 30 seconds after the COTA provides a verbal cue. Which statement represents a short-term objective to use during the **NEXT** stage of this learning process?

    1. "The child will press a switch-operated toy within 15 seconds of verbal cueing 5 out of 5 times."
    2. "The child will consistently activate a switch-operated toy without verbal cueing."
    3. "The child will actively participate in activities during one 30-minute OT session."
    4. "The child will participate in play activity using switch technology for 15-minute intervals."

15. A third grade student with ADHD has had many academic failures resulting in low self-esteem, social self-isolation, and difficulty interacting with peers during classroom activities. Which recommendation should the COTA make to the teacher to help improve the student's self-esteem and classroom performance?

    1. Allow the student to try new activities independently.
    2. Present each activity to the student in achievable steps.
    3. Involve the student in group activities frequently during the day.
    4. Encourage the student to participate in challenging activities.

16. A client who has a substance abuse disorder has been participating in a community-based OT program. The COTA feels as though the client has attained maximum benefits from a work skills group. Which action should the COTA take based on the principles of best practice?

    1. Advise the client that OT is no longer indicated.
    2. Discuss the client's status with the supervising OTR.
    3. Re-evaluate the client prior to the next group.
    4. Discharge the client from this particular group.

17. A inpatient who recently had a CVA is preparing for discharge to live alone at home. The patient has persistent edema of the affected upper extremity despite using proper positioning techniques. What task should be completed prior to the patient's discharge to promote self-management of the upper extremity edema?

    1. Fabricate a resting hand splint for the patient to wear at all times.
    2. Instruct the patient how to perform manual massage techniques.
    3. Provide the patient with a handout for preparing home paraffin baths.
    4. Arrange to loan the patient a functional electrical stimulation unit.

18. A client who has had a CVA initially required moderate verbal cues to complete oral hygiene and grooming. Now the client consistently completes these tasks independently during self-care sessions. Based on this progress, what action should the COTA take prior to the next intervention session with this client?

    1. Recommend discharge from OT.
    2. Re-evaluate functional performance.
    3. Discuss the progress with the physician.
    4. Collaborate with the OTR to review goals.

19. Which of the following sets of homemaking activities uses the greatest range of bilateral shoulder flexion and elbow extension?

    1. Ironing shirts and placing them on a hanger
    2. Washing dishes in a sink and drying pots and pans
    3. Folding sheets and hanging towels on a clothesline
    4. Dusting tabletops and vacuuming carpets

20. A COTA and OTR are collaborating on an intervention plan for an inpatient who had a recent TBI and is functioning at Level V (Confused-inappropriate, Non-agitated) on the Rancho Los Amigos scale. Which intervention environment is **MOST CONDUCIVE** for promoting initial progress toward functional goals?

    1. In the quietest section of the rehabilitation department
    2. In the therapy clinic when other therapists are treating patients
    3. In the day room near the patient's room with a group of other patients
    4. In the patient's room when family members are present

21. A COTA is scheduled to participate in a multidisciplinary discharge planning meeting for an inpatient who has amyotrophic lateral sclerosis, and is in the hospital due to a recent physical decline. Which information about the patient is **MOST IMPORTANT** for the COTA gather in preparation for the initial meeting?

    1. Vocational and leisure history
    2. Functional activities completed in OT
    3. Overview of previous outpatient services
    4. Durable medical equipment needs for ADL

22. Which data gathering process should be included in an **INITIAL** work readiness evaluation with a young adult who has mild cognitive impairment, poor attention span, and limited frustration tolerance?

    1. Vocational interest inventory
    2. Standardized gross motor assessment
    3. Job skills simulation activities
    4. Strength and endurance measurements

23. A client who has schizophrenia has recently transitioned from living at home with parents to residing in a group home. What is the **PRIMARY** reason for interviewing the client's parents as part of the information gathering process when using a cognitive disabilities approach?

    1. Learning about the client's emotional needs
    2. Determining the client's developmental stage
    3. Becoming aware of the client's unconscious conflicts
    4. Identifying the client's performance patterns

24. During which task would a stereognosis deficit secondary to a CVA be **MOST EVIDENT**?

    1. Picking up objects from a tabletop
    2. Turning on a water faucet
    3. Getting keys from a pocket
    4. Holding eating utensils

25. Which strategy provides the **MOST OBJECTIVE** information about the ADL skills of an inpatient who has had a recent CVA?

    1. Asking the nursing staff about the patient's performance
    2. Having the patient complete a self-care questionnaire
    3. Interviewing family members about the patient's preferences
    4. Observing the patient completing self-care tasks

26. A client who has multiple sclerosis works as an administrative assistant in a large corporation. Fatigue and weakness interfere with the client's ability to complete job tasks. The corporate physician is requesting a job site analysis for this client. What is the **PRIMARY** purpose of this type of analysis?

    1. Observing the client interacting with co-workers within the office environment
    2. Determining the critical work demands in relation to client needs
    3. Assessing the client's vocational interests in relation to work assignments
    4. Identifying the management's willingness to provide special accommodations

27. A COTA observes that a client who has had a CVA is having difficulty initiating motor tasks required for completing a subtest of a standardized assessment. What action should the COTA take upon making this observation?

1. Provide additional tactile cues.
2. Refer to the test protocol manual.
3. Use additional visual cues.
4. Repeat the test protocol instructions.

28. A client who has had a right CVA is participating in OT to promote independence with meal preparation. Which method provides the **MOST OBJECTIVE** information about the client's kitchen safety for stovetop cooking?

1. Talking with the client to learn their insight about potential safety issues
2. Asking the client to identify unsafe situations in a series of activity pictures
3. Interviewing the client during a cooking task regarding their safety concerns
4. Observing the client prepare a simple hot meal from a cookbook recipe

29. An inpatient who has left hemiplegia wants to be independent in bathing. Which step should the COTA complete **FIRST** to promote the patient's progress toward this goal?

1. Review one-handed bathing techniques with the patient.
2. Determine the patient's current self-care abilities.
3. Inquire about the planned discharge environment.
4. Provide instruction in the use of adaptive equipment.

30. A COTA is collaborating with an OTR to determine intervention needs for an elementary school student. Which of the following data will provide the **MOST** information about the student's current skills and abilities?

1. Physician's referral request
2. Standardized test scores
3. Classroom performance
4. Birth history

31. A student who has moderate developmental delay has been participating in school-based OT. Which information is **MOST IMPORTANT** for the COTA to provide to the supervising OTR prior to the student's upcoming re-evaluation?

1. Current cognitive abilities and verbal skills
2. Typical motor performance compared to peers
3. Performance patterns during curriculum-based activities
4. Changes in ability to participate in leisure activities

32. Which symptoms have the **MOST** impact on self-feeding for a client who has early Parkinson's disease?

    1. Joint contractures and deformities
    2. Incoordination and bradykinesia
    3. Diminished protective sensations and strength
    4. Hypertonicity and spasticity

33. One of the goals of a client in a home health setting is to increase active shoulder flexion. As part of the intervention, the client removes collectible items from wall-mounted shelves, dusts the items and the shelves, and returns the collectibles to the shelves. What is the purpose for including this task in the client's program?

    1. Simulating a variety of movement patterns
    2. Facilitating isometric muscle contractions
    3. Promoting cleanliness within the home
    4. Using purposeful activity for promoting goals

34. An elder adult who has had a CVA was admitted to an inpatient rehabilitation facility two days ago. The patient is scheduled to participate in an initial self-care session. Prior to the session the COTA learns that the patient immigrated to the United States several years ago and is living with family members. Which action should the COTA complete **INITIALLY** based on this information?

    1. Apply broad generalizations about the patient's culture to self-care activities.
    2. Gather information about the patient's cultural values regarding self-care.
    3. Initiate self-care activities based on experience with other patients.
    4. Administer a standardized evaluation to determine the patient's current function.

The following multiple-choice items are samples related to Domain Area 2:

Select and implement evidence-based interventions to support participation in areas of occupation (e.g., ADL, education, work, play, leisure, and social participation) throughout the continuum of care

35. A COTA is planning an inservice to instruct the nursing staff at a long-term care facility about safe transfer techniques. What is the **PRIMARY** objective of this type of inservice?

    1. Identifying injury risk factors and minimize hazards
    2. Reducing workers' compensation claims within the facility
    3. Complying with OSHA annual training requirements
    4. Decreasing facility liability for job-related injuries

36. What should be the **PRIMARY** focus of a wellness program for elder adults who reside in an assisted living facility?

    1. Engaging participants in a variety of health-seeking behaviors
    2. Locating community resources available for the aged population
    3. Conducting discussions about common health and mobility problems
    4. Assisting residents develop a monthly schedule of preferred activities

37. The activities director at a senior center tells the COTA that some individuals in a gourmet cooking class are finding it difficult to actively participate due to painful hands. Which modification should the COTA recommend to support participation in the class?

    1. Use pre-cut frozen vegetables in recipes.
    2. Organize food in cabinets at ergonomic heights.
    3. Use rocker knives with serrated-edge blades.
    4. Place built-up handles on utensils.

38. Which information is **MOST IMPORTANT** to include in a presentation about injury prevention for employees at a data-entry and computer software company?

    1. Symptoms associated with cumulative trauma
    2. Types of exercise to resolve painful symptoms
    3. Impact of work-related injuries on the company
    4. Methods for reducing work-related risk factors

39. The multidisciplinary team at a community-based program is developing a substance abuse relapse program. The focus of the program is to promote healthy alternatives for at-risk individuals. What is the **PRIMARY** contribution of the COTA during the initial phase of program development?

    1. Asking potential participants about past leisure interests
    2. Identifying area resources and potential barriers to participation
    3. Suggesting program objectives related to leisure skill development
    4. Determining specific outcome measures for the program

40. A client who has schizophrenia is participating in psychiatric day treatment program. During an OT group, the client admits to "forgetting" to take prescribed medications. What is the **NEXT** action that the COTA should take after discussing the importance of taking the prescription medication with the client?

    1. Contact the referring physician and report the client's noncompliance.
    2. Alert the client's family or significant other to the issue.
    3. Document the client's noncompliance and the outcome of the discussion.
    4. Have the client sign a behavioral contract agreeing to take the medication.

41. An inpatient who has congestive heart failure and now requires a wheelchair for mobility will be discharged to live in an apartment with family members. During a home visit, the COTA identifies several areas in the apartment that are not accessible by a wheelchair. What should the COTA do **NEXT** based on this information?

    1. Collaborate with the patient and family to discuss the needs.
    2. Ask the family members to rearrange the furniture for wheelchair access.
    3. Have family members notify the apartment manager of needed changes.
    4. Assess the patient's ability to ambulate short distances with a walker.

42. An adolescent who has a conduct disorder is participating in an OT group to increase socialization skills. While playing a familiar board game, the adolescent loses a turn, becomes frustrated, and demands to play something else. How should the COTA respond to the adolescent's behavior?

    1. Modify the game rules to promote success.
    2. Excuse the adolescent from the activity session.
    3. Encourage the adolescent to complete the activity.
    4. Allow the adolescent to select another activity.

43. While participating in a group gardening activity, the COTA observes that a client who has multiple sclerosis becomes extremely fatigued. What **INITIAL** action should the COTA take in response to this observation?

    1. Remind the client to use energy conservation techniques.
    2. Ask another client to assist in completing the gardening task.
    3. Discontinue the gardening activity for the day.
    4. Demonstrate gardening work-simplification techniques.

44. A school-based COTA is working with a student who has athetoid cerebral palsy with moderate extensor tone. Which method is **MOST EFFECTIVE** for inhibiting the student's extensor patterns when a caregiver is moving the student from the wheelchair to the floor?

    1. Support the student's trunk with one arm and abduct the lower extremity with the other arm.
    2. Hold the student facing forward with hips and knees flexed and neck slightly flexed.
    3. Have the student's back face the caregiver with hips and knees extended and neck slightly flexed.
    4. Position the student so the legs straddle the caregiver's hip.

45. A client is working on a needlework project for a grandchild's birthday, but is having difficulty finishing the project due to low vision from early stage cataracts. The client is scheduled for cataract surgery, but the surgery date is after the grandchild's birthday. Which compensatory technique should the COTA recommend to promote the client's ability to finish the needlework project in time for the birthday?

    1. Advise the client to use high contrast colored thread.
    2. Place the project in an adjustable frame.
    3. Reduce the amount of ambient light in the room.
    4. Provide the client with a lighted, hands-free magnifier.

46. A client who has paraplegia wants to prepare family meals independently. Which environmental modification will promote the client's safety during stovetop cooking?

    1. Positioning an angled mirror above the stove
    2. Replacing stove knobs with larger handles
    3. Using pots with extended handles
    4. Stirring hot liquids with rubber-coated, cooking utensils

47. A patient who has Alzheimer's disease attempts to elope from a nursing facility every afternoon when the nursing staff changes shift stating, "I need to go back to work." Which action is **MOST EFFECTIVE** for redirecting the patient's attention and decreasing the risk of elopement?

   1. Having the patient participate in a simple craft activity
   2. Taking the patient outside for a walk in the garden
   3. Encouraging the patient to watch television with other residents
   4. Engaging the patient in an activity reminiscent of a valued occupational role

48. Which assistive device is **MOST** useful for promoting independence with self-feeding for a client who has a complete C_6 spinal cord injury?

   1. Switch-operated feeder
   2. Mobile arm support
   3. Tenodesis splint
   4. Wrist cock-up splint

49. Which assistive device is **MOST** useful for promoting independence with self-feeding for a client who is in Stage II of Parkinson's disease?

   1. Rocker knife
   2. Weighted utensil
   3. Long-handle utensil
   4. Swivel spoon

50. A kindergarten-age student who has spastic cerebral palsy is painting while seated at a table in art class. The student can hold a paintbrush, but a dominant asymmetrical tonic neck reflex prevents the student from reaching for the paint that is located near the student's dominant side. Which technique is **MOST EFFECTIVE** for inhibiting this reflex?

   1. Placing the paint at midline in front of the student
   2. Providing the student with a paintbrush with a weighted handle
   3. Adapting the tabletop to a 45° elevated angle
   4. Having the student use a standing frame while painting

51. A COTA is recommending environmental adaptations for an individual who has rheumatoid arthritis and works in a medical laboratory. The individual reports increased pain when turning knobs and tightening specimen cup lids. Which movements are **CONTRAINDICATED** for this patient to use during these job tasks?

   1. Wrist extension
   2. MCP joint ulnar deviation
   3. Wrist ulnar deviation
   4. Composite finger extension

52. An inpatient who has an incomplete T_2 spinal cord injury is learning wheelchair transfers. The patient is able to independently transfer without assistive devices from the bed to the wheelchair, but has difficulty transferring from the wheelchair to the toilet. What should the COTA do **NEXT** as part of the transfer training program?

   1. Encourage the patient use a bedside commode instead of the bathroom toilet.
   2. Teach the patient to use a sliding board and a hydraulic lift.
   3. Complete a manual muscle test to determine the patient's triceps strength.
   4. Evaluate the difference in the height between the wheelchair and the toilet.

53. A COTA is teaching an individual who has Parkinson's disease how to transport food items in the kitchen using a walker with an attached tray. Which of the following instructions should the COTA provide to the individual during the session?

   1. Stand inside the frame of the walker and turn slowly.
   2. Turn the walker to the desired direction then move the legs.
   3. Move the walker to one side and use the counter for support.
   4. Place one hand on the counter and the other on the walker to move it.

54. One of the intervention goals for a 4-year-old child who has moderate cerebral palsy is to improve oral-motor control for eating and swallowing. Which activity should be included during the **INITIAL** phase of intervention to promote the child's lip closure and awareness of oral movement?

   1. Sipping fruit juice from a cup
   2. Blowing bubbles into the air
   3. Whistling a simple tune
   4. Sucking a flavored ice-pop

55. An individual who has chronic low back pain notes an increase in symptoms when doing laundry. Which activity represents a body mechanics technique that should be used during laundry activities to minimize the onset of symptoms?

    1. Carry one small basket of laundry at a time to the laundry area.
    2. Lift one large bundle of clothes from the washer to put into the dryer.
    3. Bend forward while loading clothes into the washer or dryer.
    4. Twist at the waist when placing clothes from the washer into the dryer.

56. A patient who had a total hip replacement two weeks ago wants to lie on the non-affected hip while sleeping. Adhering to post-surgical hip precautions, how should the patient be advised on the **BEST** positioning for sleeping?

    1. Place a pillow under both legs.
    2. Use an abduction wedge between the legs.
    3. Sleep on an air mattress.
    4. Flex the affected hip and extend the legs.

57. A client who has had a recent partial hand amputation is losing interest in attending OT, and has stopped complying with the home exercise program. Which action should be taken **INITIALLY** based on the client's behavior?

    1. Contact the client's significant others about the lack of progress.
    2. Discuss these observations and concerns with the client.
    3. Decrease the frequency and intensity of the overall intervention program.
    4. Review the treatment plan and long-term goals with the client.

58. During a woodworking group, an individual who has had a spinal cord injury complains of a pounding headache, begins to perspire, and has chills. What **INITIAL** action should the COTA take in response to the individual's symptoms?

    1. Treat the incident as a medical emergency and call for help.
    2. Transport the individual to their room to rest.
    3. Monitor the individual closely for any additional symptoms.
    4. Ask the patient about allergies to wood varnishes or stains.

59. For religious reasons, a client refuses to make decorations for a holiday party as part of a group activity. How should the COTA respond to the client's refusal?

    1. Encourage the client to respect the values of the other group participants.
    2. Suggest the client discuss reasons for refusing with a pastoral counselor.
    3. Explore the reasons for the conflict between the activity and religious beliefs.
    4. Offer an alternative group activity that is pertinent to the established goals.

60. A COTA who works at an assisted living facility is taking four residents on an outing to a restaurant. Several of the participants have hearing impairments. Which arrangement with the restaurant should the COTA make to promote socialization among the residents during the meal?

    1. Be sure there is a table located close to the kitchen so the residents are comfortable speaking loudly to each other.
    2. Reserve a table that is located in a busy section of the restaurant so loud talking will not disturb other patrons.
    3. Ask to be seated at a round dining table that will comfortably accommodate the residents.
    4. Request a table that is directly under a fluorescent overhead light so participants are able to read menus.

61. Which of the following is **MOST IMPORTANT** for the COTA to do in preparation for a self-care session with an inpatient who has COPD?

    1. Arrange ADL supplies so they are within easy reach for the patient.
    2. Make sure the patient has adequate standing tolerance to complete the entire activity.
    3. Determine the patient's preferences for supplies such as spray deodorants and talcum powder.
    4. Place a chair just outside of the bathroom door in case the patient becomes fatigued.

62. Which kitchen modification is **BEST** to recommend for a client who has reduced visual acuity and wants to remain independent with meal preparation tasks?

    1. Labeling food items in large print using high-contrast colors
    2. Using fluorescent bulbs in household light fixtures
    3. Keeping frequently used items on the countertop
    4. Replacing wooden cabinet doors with glass panels

63. A client who has had a CVA is baking cookies in OT. The COTA observes that although the client uses the correct amount of dough for each cookie, the client places the dough only on the right side of the cookie sheet before stating that the pan is ready to place in the oven. Which sensory processing deficit is this behavior **TYPICALLY** associated with?

    1. Figure-ground neglect
    2. Homonymous hemianopsia
    3. Diminished depth perception
    4. Right-left disorientation

64. A client who has mild-moderate dementia has difficulty remembering when to take a prescribed medicine. Which compensatory technique will promote this client's ability to independently take medications at the correct dosage time?

    1. Placing medications in a seven-day pill storage container at the beginning of each week
    2. Wearing a voice-message alarm that is preprogrammed to activate at specific times of the day
    3. Maintaining a medication diary that outlines a daily medication history
    4. Using a pocket day-planner that indicates which medications to take each day

65. A client who has a substance abuse disorder has been able to maintain employment, but has difficulty managing time, interacting with others, and attending to homemaking activities. What should be the **PRIMARY** goal of intervention when working with this client?

    1. Transitioning the client to a group living environment
    2. Promoting practical skills for basic personal life management
    3. Encouraging the client to participate in leisure activities with friends
    4. Teaching the client methods for reducing work-related stressors

66. Which craft material is **CONTRAINDICATED** to use for an inpatient who has cancer and has decreased platelet level due to chemotherapy medications?

    1. Burlap or yarn
    2. Water-based paints
    3. Scented markers or pens
    4. Self-opening scissors

67. Which strategy is **BEST** for promoting a positive exploration of feelings with a group of adolescents who have anorexia?

    1. Incorporate valued activities that the participants select.
    2. Pre-determine structured activities for the participants to complete.
    3. Provide challenging, multi-step, activities based on the participants' cognition.
    4. Use a variety of role-playing activities emphasizing body image.

68. A professional pianist who had a left CVA resulting in mild, right hemiparesis wants to increase strength and fine motor control of the affected extremity. Which intervention activity is the **BEST** example of a client-centered intervention for promoting progress toward this goal?

    1. Making a pinch pot using firm modeling clay
    2. Manipulating various size pegs and stringing one-inch beads
    3. Practicing a repetitive program of keyboard drills
    4. Completing therapy band exercises while listening to piano music

69. An inpatient who has schizophrenia, paranoid type, is beginning to tolerate being around several other people at the same time. Which type of group activity is **BEST** for the patient to attend to promote socialization?

    1. Values clarification
    2. Parallel task
    3. Competitive team sport
    4. Community outing

70. A client who has COPD has difficulty completing home management tasks due to increasing episodes of dyspnea and fatigue. Which of the following techniques should the client learn during the **INITIAL** phase of rehabilitation reduce the impact of these symptoms on function?

    1. Energy conservation
    2. Strengthening exercises
    3. Stress management
    4. Visual imagery

71. Which activity is **BEST** for promoting bilateral upper extremity coordinated movements for a group of children who are 3-years-old and have mild developmental delay?

    1. Rolling a large therapy ball to each other
    2. Playing dress-up to imitate action heroes
    3. Playing prone-lying scooter board games
    4. Jumping rope to music

72. What should be the **INITIAL** focus of a craft activity for a group of inpatients who have major depression?

    1. Completion of a simple project
    2. Promoting success in a valued task
    3. Participant interaction with each other
    4. Diversion from the hospital environment

73. A 5-year-old child who has moderate hypertonicity of the upper extremities is participating in OT to increase independence in dressing. Which technique is **MOST EFFECTIVE** for normalizing the child's muscle tone prior to initiating a dressing task?

    1. Bouncing the child up and down on a large therapy ball
    2. Having the child gently rock forward and backward in quadruped
    3. Using quick tapping to the spastic muscle bellies
    4. Applying heavy joint compression to both arms

74. A 9-year-old child who has moderate hemiplegia often neglects to use the affected upper extremity. Which activity is **BEST** for encouraging the child's bilateral fine motor movement patterns?

    1. Playing with a hand-held video game
    2. Tossing a beanbag at a target
    3. Playing a game of darts
    4. Drawing on a chalkboard

75. An individual who has moderate dementia and lives in an assisted living facility frequently gets lost on the way to the dining room. Which environmental modification is **MOST BENEFICIAL** for enabling the individual to independently find the way to the dining room?

    1. Painting the walls leading to the dining room with bright colors
    2. Posting simple, familiar signs along the route to the dining room
    3. Dimming overhead fluorescent lighting to create a more home-like atmosphere
    4. Providing multiple visual and auditory cues in the hallways and common areas

76. Which technique is **MOST EFFECTIVE** for a client to use for managing the symptoms of COPD during a functional task at home?

    1. Breathing out when pushing items and breathing in when pulling items
    2. Inhaling through the mouth and exhaling through the nose when lifting
    3. Taking shallow quick breaths whenever shortness of breath occurs
    4. Crossing both arms across the chest when breathing becomes difficult

77. A second grade student uses a palmar grasp whenever holding a pencil. Which intervention activity is effective for promoting a more mature pencil grasp pattern with this student?

    1. Stringing one-inch beads
    2. Finger-painting on an easel
    3. Rolling out modeling dough
    4. Cutting shapes using adapted scissors

78. A COTA is selecting activities for a first grade student who has mild visual memory deficits. Which activity is **MOST BENEFICIAL** for promoting the student's long-term visual memory storage?

    1. Creating rhymes about facts presented in a class assignment
    2. Having the student repetitively practice spelling word lists
    3. Playing follow-the-leader with the student
    4. Having the student copy patterns from a puzzle book

79. A school-age child who is blind and has severe tactile defensiveness will be participating in OT to improve sensory processing prior to learning Braille. Which activity should be included as part of the child's **INITIAL** intervention?

    1. Object identification games with vision occluded
    2. Fun activities that reinforce pre-reading concepts
    3. Drills for assigning meaning to raised dots on paper
    4. Graded play using a variety of textured materials

80. A COTA is fabricating a splint for a client who recently had a deep partial thickness burn to the dorsum of the hand. When the COTA removes the bulky dressing, the patient becomes lightheaded and begins to sweat. What **INITIAL** action should the COTA take in response to this occurrence?

    1. Break open an ammonia ampule and slowly pass it under the client's nose.
    2. Assist the client to a supine position and elevate the client's legs.
    3. Ask the client to rest their head on the table or between their knees.
    4. Moisten a cloth with cool water and hold it across the client's forehead.

81. An elder adult who has mild macular degeneration is referred to OT. The client is an avid reader but is having progressive difficulty reading a favorite magazine due to the reflective glare from the glossy paper. Which adaptation is **MOST BENEFICIAL** for supporting the client's participation in this preferred leisure activity?

   1. Using audio and large print books that are loaned from a local library
   2. Subscribing to satellite radio to be able to listen to books and news stories
   3. Directing the lighting source from behind the client's shoulder when reading
   4. Contacting publishers to see if the magazine is available with matte finish print

82. A client who has an anxiety disorder recently immigrated to the United States with a spouse and two children. The client's goal is to fully participate in family roles and routines. During a homemaking session with the client, what should the COTA do to **MOST EFFECTIVELY** assist the client in making progress toward this goal?

   1. Respect the culture and values of the client.
   2. Encourage the client to adapt to social norms of this country.
   3. Instruct the client how to use modern appliances.
   4. Teach the client about the family values system in this country.

The following multiple-choice items are samples related to Domain Area 3:
Uphold professional standards and responsibilities to promote quality in practice

83. A COTA and OTR working in a skilled nursing facility are collaborating on an initial intervention plan for an inpatient who has a hip and wrist fracture. Which information **MUST** be included in this patient's documentation to meet Medicare requirements for reimbursement of services?

   1. Expected changes joint ROM and pain level
   2. Activities that the COTA will be responsible for providing
   3. Long-term functional goals that are medically necessary
   4. Specific intervention techniques that will be used

84. An inpatient who has a complete C_7 spinal cord injury has been participating in OT for one week to increase independence in upper extremity dressing. The patient is now able to independently sit up in bed and put on a pullover shirt, but still requires caregiver assistance to get the shirt from the closet. Which statement about the patient is **BEST** to include in the "A" section of the next SOAP progress note?

   1. "The patient is learning compensatory strategies and is moving towards the long-term dressing goal as stated in the initial plan."
   2. "The patient will require assistive devices and assistance from a caregiver for most self-care tasks after discharge."
   3. "The patient wants to learn how to use additional adaptive devices for lower body dressing and bathing."
   4. "The patient is independent in upper extremity dressing from a seated position, but still needs some caregiver assistance."

85. An elderly inpatient who is recovering from pneumonia, has generalized weakness and ambulates with a cane. The patient is scheduled to begin self-care sessions. Which risk management technique should the COTA use when walking the patient from the bed to the bathroom during the initial session in the patient's room?

    1. Have the patient wear a transfer belt and use a walker.
    2. Ask a caregiver to provide additional stand-by assistance.
    3. Have the patient put on rubber-sole shoes before walking.
    4. Ask the patient to walk with a slow, shuffling gait.

86. An elderly client who had a recent wrist fracture has been attending OT 3 times per week for several weeks. The client's ROM and strength are improving, but the client is still reluctant to use the affected hand. At the end of a session, the client refuses to schedule more OT visits citing "transportation problems". What should the COTA **INITIALLY** do in this situation?

    1. Talk with the client to determine a solution.
    2. Teach the client an independent home program.
    3. Refer the client to a home health agency.
    4. Encourage scheduling a monthly reevaluation.

87. A patient who had a total knee replacement three days ago is being discharged from an acute-care facility to an inpatient rehabilitation program. Which information can be used to determine outcomes, and should be included in the OT discharge summary?

    1. Recommendations for specific treatment interventions
    2. Level of the patient's occupational function prior to hospitalization
    3. Objective information on functional goals achieved
    4. Statements about the patient's participation in goal setting

88. A client who has major depression has been participating in OT in an acute inpatient psychiatric hospital. The client is preparing for discharge and will receive follow-up services in a community mental health program. Which information related to OT intervention outcomes is **MOST IMPORTANT** to include in the client's discharge summary?

    1. Changes in job performance skills during simulated work activities
    2. Improvement in gross and fine motor skills required for ADL
    3. Subjective impressions of the client's functional independence
    4. Current self-care abilities compared to initial evaluation results

89. Which strategy is **MOST EFFECTIVE** for promoting successful outcomes of a community-based smoking cessation program for senior citizens who have early symptoms of COPD?

    1. Posting pictures showing plastic models of diseased lungs
    2. Educating participants about health risks and lifestyle changes
    3. Recommending over-the-counter nicotine substitutes
    4. Allowing time for individual counseling sessions

90. A COTA is working in an outpatient hand therapy clinic, but plans to change jobs and work in an inpatient neuro-rehabilitation setting. Which action should the COTA take as an **INITIAL** step toward developing service competency in the new job?

    1. Arrange to have close supervision whenever working with a client.
    2. Provide the OTR with a list of service competent tasks from the previous job.
    3. Learn about clinical protocols by leading a staff discussion on the topic.
    4. Ask an OTR to review and co-sign each patient contact note.

91. A school-based OTR and COTA are collaborating to evaluate a kindergarten-age student who has autism. Which task can the COTA complete as part of this data gathering process?

    1. Score a sensory integration assessment.
    2. Select developmentally-appropriate assessment tools.
    3. Analyze evaluation results.
    4. Administer a developmental skills checklist.

92. A COTA who works in an inpatient rehabilitation clinic has been assigned to supervise a newly hired therapy aide. Which information **MUST** the COTA know prior to assigning job tasks to the aide?

    1. The OT practice act guidelines for service provision
    2. The critical demands listed in the aide's job description
    3. The aide's previous experience working with patients
    4. The aide's knowledge of occupational therapy

93. Which information is **TYPICALLY** placed in the "O" section of the SOAP note?

    1. Long-term functional goals
    2. Measurable data from ongoing treatment
    3. Statements made by patient and/or family
    4. Judgments a client's functional limitations

94. Which information should be evident in client contact notes in order to justify the need for additional OT services to a client's insurance company?

    1. Subjective reports of progress in therapy
    2. Progress as it relates to the initial functional goals
    3. Comments on anticipated function at discharge
    4. Rate of progress as compared to other patients

95. A COTA who works in a psychiatric facility is supervising a craft group for inpatients who have schizophrenia and are functioning at Allen Cognitive Level 3 (Manual actions). What is **MOST IMPORTANT** for the COTA to do prior to the end of the session?

    1. Ensure that equipment and supplies used during the session are collected and counted.
    2. Have the patients use an antibacterial solution to wipe clean all of the tables and countertops.
    3. Label all of the projects so they can be easily identified at the beginning of the next session.
    4. Have the patients sign an attendance roster.

96. A COTA is teaching compensatory techniques for facial shaving to a client who has mild choreiform movements of the upper extremity. Which of the following is the **BEST** example of incorporating universal precautions into the task?

    1. Using a straight-edge razor that can be cleaned with alcohol
    2. Having the client practice with an electric shaver borrowed from the OT self-care room
    3. Having the client bring in an electric shaver to use during each session
    4. Asking the client to purchase a bag of disposable straight-edge razors

97. A COTA is working in a skilled nursing facility that operates under Medicare regulations. Which information **MUST** the COTA document after each intervention session to meet reimbursement requirements of the prospective payment system (PPS)?

    1. The patient's response to specific treatment techniques
    2. The supplies and equipment used during the session
    3. The total number of minutes spent treating the patient
    4. The day and time of the next scheduled treatment session

98. A newly certified COTA is working in a large rehabilitation clinic where dynamic splints are fabricated routinely. The COTA received basic splinting instruction in school, yet feels the need for further training. What action is necessary for establishing service competency in this area?

1. Referring to a textbook picture of the splint when fabricating a splint for a client
2. Arranging for supervision and participate in structured learning about splinting
3. Making a checklist of key tips to use when fabricating dynamic splints
4. Reviewing school notes and read journal articles about splinting

99. A COTA is preparing to give a presentation for an arthritis support group. Which presentation method will **MOST EFFECTIVELY** communicate the role of occupational therapy in assisting individuals who have this disease?

1. Describing the OT assessments typically used with individuals who have arthritis
2. Discussing OT interventions and service options for individuals who have arthritis
3. Simulating an OT session using one of the participants as an example
4. Demonstrating exercise programs for individuals who have arthritis

100. A COTA who is employed by the state department of vocational rehabilitation is asked to give a presentation to a parent group on the role of OT in the program. Which method is **MOST EFFECTIVE** for communicating the value of OT to this audience?

1. Discussing how task skills and work behaviors impact student employability
2. Describing the disabilities of the students enrolled in the program
3. Demonstrating assistive technology used for improving performance
4. Outlining parental responsibility in helping their children obtain employment

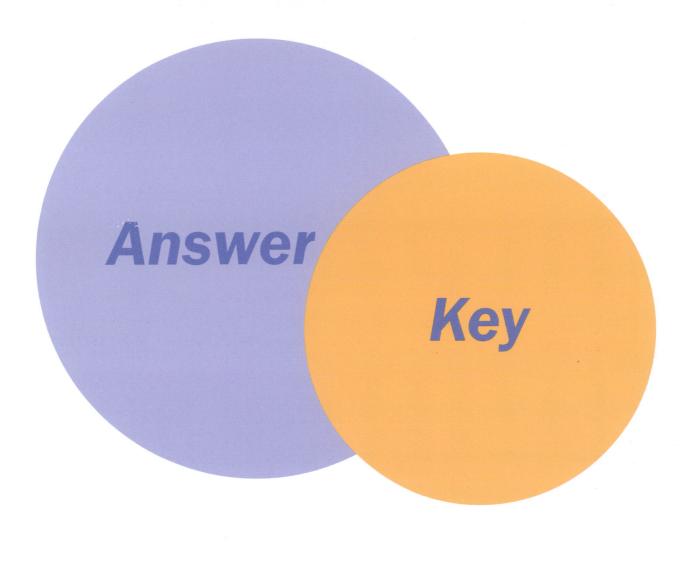

Answer Key

Answer Key for the COTA Study Guide Sample Items

1-3	26-2	51-2	76-1
2-4	27-2	52-4	77-1
3-2	28-4	53-1	78-1
4-2	29-2	54-2	79-4
5-2	30-3	55-1	80-2
6-1	31-3	56-2	81-3
7-1	32-2	57-2	82-1
8-2	33-4	58-1	83-3
9-2	34-2	59-4	84-1
10-4	35-1	60-3	85-3
11-2	36-1	61-1	86-1
12-2	37-4	62-1	87-3
13-1	38-4	63-2	88-4
14-1	39-3	64-2	89-2
15-2	40-1	65-2	90-1
16-2	41-1	66-4	91-4
17-2	42-3	67-1	92-1
18-4	43-3	68-3	93-2
19-3	44-2	69-2	94-2
20-4	45-4	70-1	95-1
21-4	46-1	71-1	96-3
22-1	47-4	72-2	97-3
23-4	48-3	73-2	98-2
24-3	49-2	74-1	99-2
25-4	50-1	75-2	100-1

1. **Correct Answer: 3**

   Demonstration of service competency should be achieved before independently administering a manual muscle test to a client.

   Incorrect Answers:

   1: This does not establish competence or skill level.

   2: The COTA does not have service competency to perform the test

   4: This can be used as a part of establishing competency, only if the colleague is competent in the testing procedures and the OTR is the practitioner who ultimately determines competency.

   Reference: Early, M. B. (2006). *Physical Dysfunction Practice Skills for the Occupational Therapy Assistant* (2nd ed.). St. Louis, MO: Elsevier Mosby, Inc. Page 139.

2. **Correct Answer: 4**

   This type of survey focuses the clients' perspective about their occupational performance.

   Incorrect Answers:

   1 ,2, 3: This type of information is not gathered in an occupational performance measure.

   Reference: Early, M. B. (2006). *Physical Dysfunction Practice Skills for the Occupational Therapy Assistant* (2nd ed.). St. Louis, MO: Elsevier Mosby, Inc. Pages 585-586.

3. **Correct Answer: 2**

   The primary role of the COTA is to make recommendations about environmental adaptations to enable the individual to access toileting facilities safely and independently. In addition, the COTA can advise on clothing adaptations and activities to improve fine motor coordination to facilitate successful clothing management.

   Incorrect Answers:

   1, 3, 4: The COTA may contribute to discussions on these topics, but it is not the primary role of a COTA.

   Reference: Byers-Connon, S., Lohman, H., Padilla, R. L. (2004). *Occupational Therapy with Elders: Strategies for the COTA* (2nd ed.). St. Louis, MO: Elsevier Mosby, Inc. Page 229.

4. **Correct Answer: 2**

   IEP reviews must be done on an annual basis. The COTA is responsible for reporting the progress in school-related activities that a student has made over the year.

   Incorrect Answers:

   1: Reporting about age-appropriate leisure activities is not related to performance during school.

   3: Although the OTR typically considers this information when interpreting standardized assessment scores, it is not generally something that the COTA reports during an IEP review

   4: These areas are most often addressed by a speech and language pathologist.

   Reference: Solomon, J. W. & O'Brien, J. C. (2006). *Pediatric Skills for Occupational Therapy Assistants* (2nd ed.). St. Louis, MO: Elsevier Mosby, Inc. Pages 62-63.

SECTION 5

Sample Items

5. *Correct Answer: 2*

Having the patient involved in decisions and setting goals is the key fundamental of the client-centered approach.

Incorrect Answers:

1, 3, 4: These do not reflect the **PRIMARY** purpose for writing client-centered goals.

Reference: Early, M. B. (2006). *Physical Dysfunction Practice Skills for the Occupational Therapy Assistant* (2nd ed.). St. Louis, MO: Elsevier Mosby, Inc. Pages 72-73.

Pendleton, H. M. & Schultz-Krohn, W. (2006). *Pedretti's Occupational Therapy: Practice Skills for Physical Dysfunction* (6th ed.). St. Louis, MO: Elsevier Mosby, Inc. Page 115.

6. *Correct Answer: 1*

The purpose of the questionnaire is to engage the individual in identifying areas of strengths and weaknesses that can be used in setting goals.

Incorrect Answers:

2: Completing a questionnaire does not facilitate socialization.
3: Responding to this questionnaire does not mean that the participants want to address their issues during a group.
4: Evaluating an individual's self-assessment skills is not the focus of this type of group.

Reference: Early, M. B. (2009). *Mental Health Concepts and Techniques for the Occupational Therapy Assistant* (4th ed.). Baltimore, MD: Wolters Kluwer - Lippincott Williams & Wilkins. Pages 448-449,543.

7. *Correct Answer: 1*

Low vision can impact an individual's functional performance in a variety of ways. It is important to identify individual needs prior to implementing new procedures or making environmental changes.

Incorrect Answers:

2, 3, 4: These are generic modifications and are not based on specific needs of the residents.

Reference: Byers-Connon, S., Lohman, H., Padilla, R. L. (2004). *Occupational Therapy with Elders: Strategies for the COTA* (2nd ed.). St. Louis, MO: Elsevier Mosby, Inc. Pages 201-203, 210-211.

8. *Correct Answer: 2*

The patient's ability to follow through with a self-directed program impacts functional outcomes and is **MOST IMPORTANT** to consider.

Incorrect Answers:

1: A detailed rationale for providing a home program is not necessary, although the client should have a general idea that the program is a means to a functional goal.
3: Demonstrating the task is more important that verbalizing the steps.
4: This is useful information to consider when providing a home exercise program, but is not as important; especially if the client is able to follow-through independently.

Reference: Early, M. B. (2006). *Physical Dysfunction Practice Skills for the Occupational Therapy Assistant* (2nd ed.). St. Louis, MO: Elsevier Mosby, Inc. Pages 187-188.

9. *Correct Answer: 2*

Instructing the patient's family on strategies to cope with the patient's functional decline is an important role of the COTA in the discharge planning process. Because the patient exhibits moderate to severely moderate decline, it is essential that supervision be provided. Family members are consistently present and familiar to the patient and least likely to interrupt familiar routines.

Incorrect Answers:

1: The patient's family may choose to have an aide assist in the care or obtain respite care; however, the most appropriate recommendation is to first instruct the family and allow them to make the decision about additional help.

3: At this stage, the patient will be unable to complete self-care tasks independently.

4: Instructing the family about medication compliance is not the focus of OT during the discharge planning process.

Reference: Early, M. B. (2006). *Physical Dysfunction Practice Skills for the Occupational Therapy Assistant* (2nd ed.). St. Louis, MO: Elsevier Mosby, Inc. Pages 523-524.

Pendleton, H. M. & Schultz-Krohn, W. (2006). *Pedretti's Occupational Therapy: Practice Skills for Physical Dysfunction* (6th ed.). St. Louis, MO: Elsevier Mosby, Inc. Pages 883-884.

10. *Correct Answer: 4*

Client-centered practice encourages self-direction through meaningful activities. Asking open-ended questions encourage the patient's active participation and input.

Incorrect Answers:

1, 2, 3: These recommendations are not based on the patient's input.

Reference: Early, M. B. (2009). *Mental Health Concepts and Techniques for the Occupational Therapy Assistant* (4th ed.). Baltimore, MD: Wolters Kluwer - Lippincott Williams & Wilkins. Pages 38-39.

11. *Correct Answer: 2*

By instructing the resident and nursing staff on proper positioning, the COTA is educating the primary individuals responsible for splint application.

Incorrect Answers:

1: Family members may not visit residents in the facility frequently enough to assure close monitoring of splint use.

3: While it is important to understand the consequences of incorrectly used equipment, this does not teach the staff how to correctly apply splints.

4: It is impractical to provide frequent follow-up care in splint use. It is usually the role of the restorative staff to maintain correct splint use.

Reference: Coppard, B.M. & Lohman, H. (2008). *Introduction to Splinting: A Clinical Reasoning and Problem-Solving Approach* (3rd ed.). St. Louis, MO: Elsevier Mosby, Inc. Page 103.

Radomski, M.V. & Trombly-Latham, C. A. (2008). *Occupational Therapy for Physical Dysfunction* (6th ed.). Baltimore, MD: Wolters Kluwer -Lippincott Williams & Wilkins. Page 473.

12. Correct Answer: 2

Memory deficits and impulsivity may compromise the individual's safety during bathing tasks. A caregiver should provide stand-by assistance in order to reduce safety risk.

Incorrect Answers:

1: The individual should not stand when taking a shower.

3: A long-handle reacher and bath mitt may be helpful, but these do not maximize safety and may present a safety risk for individuals who have cognitive deficits and impulsivity.

4: Stepping onto a bath towel may cause a fall risk.

Reference: Early, M. B. (2006). *Physical Dysfunction Practice Skills for the Occupational Therapy Assistant* (2nd ed.). St. Louis, MO: Elsevier Mosby, Inc. Page 507.

13. Correct Answer: 1

Short-term goals must be objective, achievable, measurable, and contain a timeframe for completion. A client who has Guillain-Barré syndrome needs to increase functional strength gradually to prevent relapse.

Incorrect Answers:

2: Use of proper body mechanics is important, but the statement does not reflect a short-term goal that is achievable during the next phase of rehabilitation.

3: This goal does not contain a timeframe for completion.

4: This is too general for a short-term goal and not directly related to the goal of being able to lift an infant.

Reference: Early, M. B. (2006). *Physical Dysfunction Practice Skills for the Occupational Therapy Assistant* (2nd ed.). St. Louis, MO: Elsevier Mosby, Inc. Pages 91, 72-73.

14. Correct Answer: 1

Short-term goals are based on expected improvements in performance components. Short-term goals should be achievable, objective, and reasonable.

Incorrect Answers:

2, 3, 4: These goals have subjective components and are not reasonable short-term goals.

Reference: Early, M. B. (2006). *Physical Dysfunction Practice Skills for the Occupational Therapy Assistant* (2nd ed.). St. Louis, MO: Elsevier Mosby, Inc. Pages 72-73, 91.

15. Correct Answer: 2

Breaking tasks into smaller, achievable steps, will promote success. This will help to build self-esteem and enhance classroom performance.

Incorrect Answers:

1: Letting the student attempt activities without giving instructions sets the student up for failure. Anxiety and self-doubt may inhibit the client's ability to initiate the task independently.

3: Changing activities frequently does not allow time for the student to completely master a skill.

4: Challenging activities may result in frustration and promote a fear of failure.

Reference: Sladyk, K. & Ryan, S. (2005). *Occupational Therapy Assistant Principles: Principles, Practice Issues, and Techniques* (4th ed.). Thorofare, NJ: SLACK, Inc. Pages 189-190.

Early, M. B. (2006). *Physical Dysfunction Practice Skills for the Occupational Therapy Assistant* (2nd ed.). St. Louis, MO: Elsevier Mosby, Inc. Page 140.

16. *Correct Answer: 2*

It is best practice for the COTA to collaborate with the OTR prior to changing the intervention plan or discontinuing OT services.

Incorrect Answers:

1, 3, 4: Discontinuing OT, re-evaluating the client, or advising the client not to attend a group are decisions that the OTR should make with input from the COTA.

Reference: Early, M. B. (2006). *Physical Dysfunction Practice Skills for the Occupational Therapy Assistant* (2nd ed.). St. Louis, MO: Elsevier Mosby, Inc. Pages 64, 76.

17. *Correct Answer: 2*

Manual massage is the most effective edema control technique for a patient who resides alone.

Incorrect Answers:

1: Splinting the hand at all times is contraindicated.

3: Paraffin is primarily used to decrease stiffness and relieve pain. Additionally, use of a home unit may present a safety hazard for this patient.

4: Functional electrical stimulation unit is primarily used on specific muscles as an orthotic substitution or to facilitate a movement.

Reference: Early, M. B. (2006). *Physical Dysfunction Practice Skills for the Occupational Therapy Assistant* (2nd ed.). St. Louis, MO: Elsevier Mosby, Inc. Page 592.

18. *Correct Answer: 4*

The COTA may identify the need for change to the treatment process. Any changes made to the treatment plan and goals should be done in collaboration with the OTR.

Incorrect Answers:

1: The OTR is responsible for discontinuing OT services.

2: A full re-evaluation is not indicated at this stage of treatment.

3: It is not necessary for the COTA to discuss this progress with the physician.

Reference: Early, M. B. (2006). *Physical Dysfunction Practice Skills for the Occupational Therapy Assistant* (2nd ed.). St. Louis, MO: Elsevier Mosby, Inc. Pages 64-65.

19. *Correct Answer: 3*

From the list provided, this set of homemaking tasks requires the **GREATEST** amount of bilateral shoulder flexion and elbow extension.

Incorrect Answers:

1: Ironing shirts does not promote bilateral ROM; although placing clothes on a hanger is inherently bilateral, it does not require a full range of shoulder flexion and elbow extension.

2: These homemaking activities have some bilateral components but do not require the greatest amount of shoulder flexion and elbow extension.

4: Although these homemaking activities may be graded to include some bilateral components, they do not require the greatest amount of the motions indicated.

Reference: Early, M. B. (2006). *Physical Dysfunction Practice Skills for the Occupational Therapy Assistant* (2nd ed.). St. Louis, MO: Elsevier Mosby, Inc. Pages 671-672.

20. Correct Answer: 4

Family members should be included in the patient's OT intervention process from the beginning of treatment. The patient's room is **MOST CONDUCIVE** for promoting progress because it provides the least distractions and is most familiar to the patient.

Incorrect Answers:

1: A quiet area in the rehabilitation department may still have multiple distractions. The patient's unfamiliarity with this area may further confuse the patient.

2, 3: These environments may be over-stimulating for the patient and may increase the patient's agitation and confusion.

Reference: Early, M. B. (2006). *Physical Dysfunction Practice Skills for the Occupational Therapy Assistant* (2ⁿᵈ ed.). St. Louis, MO: Elsevier Mosby, Inc. Pages 504-505

21. Correct Answer: 4

ALS is a progressive degenerative neuromuscular disease. Disease progression is rapid resulting in significant mobility deficits, and eventual paralysis. Information about the home environment is **MOST IMPORTANT** given the likely need for home modifications, durable medical equipment, and assistive devices.

Incorrect Answers:

1: Issues regarding vocational history can be addressed on an outpatient basis, and would not impact discharge plans.

2: It is unnecessary to inform the team of specific OT activities.

3: The primary focus of the initial discharge planning process is on the patient's functional performance in the home environment. Previous outpatient services are not critical to the patient's current discharge plans.

Reference: Early, M. B. (2006). *Physical Dysfunction Practice Skills for the Occupational Therapy Assistant* (2ⁿᵈ ed.). St. Louis, MO: Elsevier Mosby, Inc. Pages 76-77, 520.

22. Correct Answer: 1

Information gathered about an individual's vocational interests should be included in the INITIAL work readiness evaluation, and used as the basis for further evaluation and intervention planning.

Incorrect Answers:

2, 3, 4: If the individual's vocational interests are not identified initially, the COTA will not be able to select the best assessments to determine the physical capabilities and job readiness skills needed for a specific job or vocation.

Reference: Early, M. B. (2009). *Mental Health Concepts and Techniques for the Occupational Therapy Assistant* (4ᵗʰ ed.). Baltimore, MD: Wolters Kluwer - Lippincott Williams & Wilkins. Pages 515 - 516.

23. *Correct Answer: 4*

The **PRIMARY** reason for interviewing the parents is to identify the client's typical performance patterns to include safety issues, current skills and abilities, and functional limitations due to the cognitive disability or chronic mental illness. This information is important for facilitating the client's transition from a supervised home environment to a group home setting.

Incorrect Answers:

1, 2, 3: Once performance patterns are identified, the other areas can be explored as indicated to promote engagement in occupationally relevant activities.

Reference: Bruce, M. & Borg, B. (2002). *Psychosocial Frames of Reference: Core for Occupation-based Practice* (3rd ed.). Thorofare, NJ: SLACK, Inc. Page 244.

Early, M. B. (2009). *Mental Health Concepts and Techniques for the Occupational Therapy Assistant* (4th ed.). Baltimore, MD: Wolters Kluwer - Lippincott Williams & Wilkins. Pages 82-91.

24. *Correct Answer: 3*

Stereognosis is the ability to recognize objects by touch with vision occluded. An individual who has deficits in stereognosis is not able to recognize keys without using visual cues.

Incorrect Answers:

1, 2, 4: The vision is not occluded in any of these functional tasks. Therefore, the individual must use visual cues to perform these activities.

Reference: Early, M. B. (2006). *Physical Dysfunction Practice Skills for the Occupational Therapy Assistant* (2nd ed.). St. Louis, MO: Elsevier Mosby, Inc. Pages 168-169.

25. *Correct Answer: 4*

Observing the patient will provide the **MOST OBJECTIVE** and measurable information regarding the patient's actual functional level.

Incorrect Answers:

1, 3: Although nursing personnel and family members are sources of some information, observation of the patient's actual performance will provide the most objective information.

2:   A questionnaire may or may not reflect the patient's actual functional level and reporting may be affected by communication, cognitive, or perceptual deficits.

Reference: Early, M. B. (2006). *Physical Dysfunction Practice Skills for the Occupational Therapy Assistant* (2nd ed.). St. Louis, MO: Elsevier Mosby, Inc. Pages 467-468.

26. *Correct Answer: 2*

The **PRIMARY** purpose of this type of analysis is to observe the client performing job tasks in a natural environment. This will provide objective information for determining the impact of the disease in relation to the critical demands of the job.

Incorrect Answers:

1, 3: These do not address the physical demands of the job that are most affected by the disease process.

4:   Special accommodations are mandatory as outlined in the ADA.

Reference: Early, M. B. (2006). *Physical Dysfunction Practice Skills for the Occupational Therapy Assistant* (2nd ed.). St. Louis, MO: Elsevier Mosby, Inc. Pages 349-350.

27. Correct Answer: 2

When administrating a standardized assessment, the established administration procedures must be strictly followed. If the protocols are not followed, the assessment results are not reliable.

Incorrect Answers:

1, 3, 4: When administering a standardized assessment, the OT practitioner may not alter or modify the test protocols, as this would alter the reliability of the assessment.

Reference: Early, M. B. (2006). *Physical Dysfunction Practice Skills for the Occupational Therapy Assistant* (2nd ed.). St. Louis, MO: Elsevier Mosby, Inc. Pages 68-69.

28. Correct Answer: 4

Directly observing the client prepare a hot meal provides the **MOST OBJECTIVE** method for identifying the client's attention to kitchen safety during a variety of related sub-tasks.

Incorrect Answers:

1: Clients who have had a CVA may have altered insight about current abilities.

2: An evaluation using photographs of household safety situations is not as reliable as actually observing the client performing a task.

3: Interviewing the client during a cooking task may be unsafe. A client may verbalize concerns, but not incorporate them in the actual activity.

Reference: Sladyk, K. & Ryan, S. (2005). *Ryan's Occupational Therapy Assistant: Principles, Practice Issues, and Techniques* (4th ed.). Thorofare, NJ: SLACK, Inc. Pages 319-320.

29. Correct Answer: 2

Assessment of the patient's current functional skill level is required **FIRST** to determine the durable medical equipment, assistive devices and instructions necessary to promote independence in bathing.

Incorrect Answers:

1, 4: Instructing adaptive bathing techniques and use of assistive equipment should begin after the initial assessment.

3: The patient's discharge environment will be influenced by the skills acquired and level of independence in self-care attained during the rehabilitation program.

Reference: Byers-Connon, S., Lohman, H., Padilla, R. L. (2004). *Occupational Therapy with Elders: Strategies for the COTA* (2nd ed.). St. Louis, MO: Elsevier Mosby, Inc. Page 245.

30. *Correct Answer: 3*

Information about and observation of the student's classroom performance provides the MOST information about the student's skills, abilities, and occupational performance needs as a student.

Incorrect Answers:

1: A physician referral is typically not necessary to initiate school-based OT intervention.

2: Standardized test scores may provide information about student's strengths and weaknesses, but they do not specifically address classroom performance, and cannot replace observation in the student's environment.

4: The student's diagnosis can provide information about possible deficits, but does not provide objective information related to the student's occupational performance needs.

Reference: Solomon, J. W. & O'Brien, J. C. (2006). *Pediatric Skills for Occupational Therapy Assistants* (2nd ed.). St. Louis, MO: Elsevier Mosby, Inc. Pages 55-56.

Case-Smith, J. (2001). *Occupational Therapy for Children* (4th ed.). St. Louis, MO: Elsevier Mosby, Inc. Page 760.

31. *Correct Answer: 3*

In a school-based setting, it is **MOST IMPORTANT** to communicate the student's progress related to curriculum-based activities.

Incorrect Answers:

1: The student's cognitive abilities and verbal skills are not the best indicator of overall performance in a school setting.

2: The performance of peers does not provide the information related to the student's functional goals in a school setting.

4: Leisure skill progress may not be directly related to academic performance.

Reference: Solomon, J. W. & O'Brien, J. C. (2006). *Pediatric Skills for Occupational Therapy Assistants* (2nd ed.). St. Louis, MO: Elsevier Mosby, Inc. Page 62.

32. *Correct Answer: 2*

The initial stage of Parkinson's disease is typically characterized by bradykinesia and incoordination. These symptoms will have the **MOST** impact on the client's ability to self-feed.

Incorrect Answers:

1, 3, 4: These are not symptoms typically associated with the initial stages of Parkinson's disease.

Reference: Early, M. B. (2006). *Physical Dysfunction Practice Skills for the Occupational Therapy Assistant* (2nd ed.). St. Louis, MO: Elsevier Mosby, Inc. Pages 516-517.

33. *Correct Answer:* 4

This activity promotes goal attainment through the use of meaningful tasks that have an inherent purpose.

Incorrect Answers:

1, 2: Although simulated and isometric activities alone may assist with goal attainment, they do not describe the activity presented in the scenario.

3: Although cleanliness in the home may be achieved during this activity, it is not part of the goal presented in the scenario.

Reference: Early, M. B. (2006). *Physical Dysfunction Practice Skills for the Occupational Therapy Assistant* (2nd ed.). St. Louis, MO: Elsevier Mosby, Inc. Pages 209-210.

34. *Correct Answer:* 2

Information about the patient's cultural values should be used to guide intervention plans and activities.

Incorrect Answers:

1, 3: These options may result in false assumptions and stereotypic bias regarding the patient's culture.

4: Many standardized OT evaluation tools do not have cross-cultural validity. Therefore, the norms can not be used to report evaluation results.

Reference: Early, M. B. (2006). *Physical Dysfunction Practice Skills for the Occupational Therapy Assistant* (2nd ed.). St. Louis, MO: Elsevier Mosby, Inc. Pages 187-188.

35. *Correct Answer:* 1

In-service training as a prevention strategy benefits both staff and clients. Identifying risk factors and reducing hazards will decrease the likelihood of work-related injuries during patient transfers.

Incorrect Answers:

2, 3, 4: These should not be the primary reason for offering nursing staff in-service training on transfer techniques.

Reference: Early, M. B. (2006). *Physical Dysfunction Practice Skills for the Occupational Therapy Assistant* (2nd ed.). St. Louis, MO: Elsevier Mosby, Inc. Pages 197-198, 312-313.

36. *Correct Answer:* 1

Wellness programs focus on promoting health-seeking behaviors and encouraging activities that promote life satisfaction.

Incorrect Answers:

2, 4: These choices are not the **PRIMARY** focus of a wellness program.

3: This choice does not emphasize wellness.

Reference: Early, M. B. (2006). *Physical Dysfunction Practice Skills for the Occupational Therapy Assistant* (2nd ed.). St. Louis, MO: Elsevier Mosby, Inc. Pages 194-195.

37. *Correct Answer: 4*

Built-up handles support participation through joint protection.

Incorrect Answers:

1: Frozen vegetables typically are not used in gourmet meal preparation recipes

2: Food and cooking items should be placed on the countertop so the individuals do not have to reach into a cabinet.

3: A rocker knife is typically used by individuals who have use of only one hand.

Reference: Byers-Connon, S., Lohman, H., Padilla, R. L. (2004). *Occupational Therapy with Elders: Strategies for the COTA* (2nd ed.). St. Louis, MO: Elsevier Mosby, Inc. Page 294.

38. *Correct Answer: 4*

The most effective method for preventing work-related injuries is to educate employees about work-related risk factors.

Incorrect Answers:

1, 3: This information is beneficial to the company management, but not to the general employee population.

2: This information is most beneficial to individuals who are being treated for a specific injury.

Reference: Early, M. B. (2006). *Physical Dysfunction Practice Skills for the Occupational Therapy Assistant* (2nd ed.). St. Louis, MO: Elsevier Mosby, Inc. Pages 352-353.

39. *Correct Answer: 3*

OT for individuals attending a substance abuse program emphasizes improving function and providing skill development.

Incorrect Answers:

1: This choice focuses on past habits that may have contributed to unhealthy lifestyles.

2, 4: These choices are not a primary role of the COTA in this type of program development process.

Reference: Early, M. B. (2009). *Mental Health Concepts and Techniques for the Occupational Therapy Assistant* (4th ed.). Baltimore, MD: Wolters Kluwer - Lippincott Williams & Wilkins. Page 161.

40. *Correct Answer: 1*

The physician needs to know that the client is noncompliant. Abruptly stopping medication can result in physical and psychological consequences.

Incorrect Answers:

2: The client's family cannot be notified unless the client has signed a consent form.

3: Documenting the client's noncompliance with the medication should be done after contacting the physician.

4: A behavioral contract for medication compliance should be done under the direction of the physician.

Reference: Early, M. B. (2009). *Mental Health Concepts and Techniques for the Occupational Therapy Assistant* (4th ed.). Baltimore, MD: Wolters Kluwer - Lippincott Williams & Wilkins. Pages 493-494.

SECTION 5

Sample Items

41. Correct Answer: 1

The COTA should collaborate with the patient and relevant others in order to prioritize the patient's needs.

Incorrect Answers:

2, 3: Collaboration with the patient and family should be done prior to making changes or recommending changes to the apartment manager.

4: It is not within the COTA scope of practice to assess ambulation.

Reference: Early, M. B. (2006). *Physical Dysfunction Practice Skills for the Occupational Therapy Assistant* (2nd ed.). St. Louis, MO: Elsevier Mosby, Inc. Pages 242-244.

42. Correct Answer: 3

Encouraging the adolescent to complete the activity sets appropriate limits and teaches the adolescent to deal with frustration in a social setting with peers.

Incorrect Answers:

1: Modifying the game rules does not promote social skills in a peer group.

2: Excusing the adolescent from the activity would only reinforce inappropriate behavior.

4: Switching to another activity would not help the adolescent deal with losing and would disrupt the group.

Reference: Case-Smith, J. (2001). *Occupational Therapy for Children* (4th ed.). St. Louis, MO: Mosby, Inc. Page 443.

43. Correct Answer: 3

The COTA should **INITIALLY** stop the activity for the day and allow the patient to rest. Extreme fatigue can trigger an exacerbation of multiple sclerosis.

Incorrect Answers:

1, 4: Client's should use energy conservation and work simplification as fatigue management techniques to minimize the onset of fatigue.

2: This may help with activity completion, but does not promote fatigue management.

Reference: Early, M. B. (2006). *Physical Dysfunction Practice Skills for the Occupational Therapy Assistant* (2nd ed.). St. Louis, MO: Elsevier Mosby, Inc. Page 513.

44. Correct Answer: 2

Flexion of the affected extremities and trunk is **MOST EFFECTIVE** for inhibiting extensor tone. Facing the student away from the caregiver enables the caregiver to position the student using good body mechanics.

Incorrect Answers:

1, 3: These positions contribute to increased extensor tone during the transfer.

4: Positioning the student in this manner does not provide adequate hip and knee flexion to inhibit extensor tone.

Reference: Solomon, J. W. & O'Brien, J. C. (2006). *Pediatric Skills for Occupational Therapy Assistants* (2nd ed.). St. Louis, MO: Elsevier Mosby, Inc. Page 223.

45. *Correct Answer: 4*

In the early stage of cataract development, a magnifier can be a helpful device to compensate for visual acuity that is inadequate to perform the sewing task.

Incorrect Answers:

1: Changing the type of thread is not realistic, since the client has already started the project.

2: This does not impact the client's ability to see the work area.

3: This would not improve the clarity of the blurred vision for completing this project.

Reference: Byers-Connon, S., Lohman, H., Padilla, R. L. (2004). *Occupational Therapy with Elders: Strategies for the COTA* (2nd ed.). St. Louis, MO: Elsevier Mosby, Inc. Pages 203-204.

Scheiman, M., Scheiman, M. & Whittaker, S. (2007). *Low Vision Rehabilitation: A Practical Guide for Occupational Therapists*. Thorofare, NJ: SLACK, Inc. Pages 70, 207-208.

46. *Correct Answer: 1*

A client who has paraplegia depends on a wheelchair for mobility. When preparing meals while seated in a wheelchair, it is difficult to see contents of pots and pans on the stovetop. Placing a mirror over the stove enables the client to see food as it is cooking, and to determine the temperature from observation. The mirror also provides visual feedback when stirring food.

Incorrect Answers:

2: Larger stove knobs would be useful for someone who has impaired vision or arthritis.

3: Smaller pans are more manageable to lift; however, reaching across burners is not as safe as using the front burners on the stove.

4: Upper extremities are not affected by paraplegia; therefore, weighted utensils are not indicated.

Reference: Early, M. B. (2006). *Physical Dysfunction Practice Skills for the Occupational Therapy Assistant* (2nd ed.). St. Louis, MO: Elsevier Mosby, Inc. Page 267.

47. *Correct Answer: 4*

"Sun-downing", plus the disruptions surrounding a shift change, can cause agitation and confusion to a patient who has Alzheimer's. Engaging the patient in an activity reminiscent of an occupational role is **MOST EFFECTIVE** for redirecting the patient during this time of the day.

Incorrect Answers:

1, 2, 3: These answers are not related to this patient's prior interest/occupation.

Reference: Byers-Connon, S., Lohman, H., Padilla, R. L. (2004). *Occupational Therapy with Elders: Strategies for the COTA* (2nd ed.). St. Louis, MO: Elsevier Mosby, Inc. Pages 257-258.

SECTION 5

Sample Items

48. *Correct Answer: 3*

A client who has a C_6 spinal cord injury typically has innervation of the radial wrist extensors. This will allow a weak tenodesis grasp. A tenodesis splint enables the client to transfer power of active wrist extension to enable a stronger pinch. This is **MOST** useful for enabling the client to hold eating utensils.

Incorrect Answers:

1: This will assist clients who have no functional use of the upper extremities.

2: A mobile arm support is used to substitute for weak proximal upper extremity strength and absent finger function.

4: A wrist cock-up splint will stabilize the wrist and interfere with the client's ability to use a functional tenodesis grip.

Reference: Early, M. B. (2006). *Physical Dysfunction Practice Skills for the Occupational Therapy Assistant* (2nd ed.). St. Louis, MO: Elsevier Mosby, Inc. Pages 536-537.

Radomski, M.V. & Trombly-Latham, C. A. (2008). *Occupational Therapy for Physical Dysfunction* (6th ed.). Baltimore, MD: Wolters Kluwer -Lippincott Williams & Wilkins. Pages 1189, 1206.

49. *Correct Answer: 2*

Clients who are in Stage II of Parkinson's disease typically have upper extremity intention tremors, the weighted fork may help to reduce these.

Incorrect Answers:

1: The primary purpose of a right-angled knife is to provide joint protection when cutting food, and would not impact the tremors.

3: Extending the length of a utensil would increase the degree of tremor.

4: The client would not be able to keep a swivel spoon steady and the spoon, although replacing limited supination, does not reduce the effects of tremors.

Reference: Early, M. B. (2006). *Physical Dysfunction Practice Skills for the Occupational Therapy Assistant* (2nd ed.). St. Louis, MO: Elsevier Mosby, Inc. Pages 253-254.

50. *Correct Answer: 1*

Head movements to either side can trigger the ATNR. Placing the paint in front of the student is **MOST EFFECTIVE** for minimizing side-to-side head movements.

Incorrect Answers:

2:   Adding weight does not inhibit the ATNR.

3, 4: The student would still have to reach for the paint; triggering the ATNR.

Reference: Solomon, J. W. & O'Brien, J. C. (2006). *Pediatric Skills for Occupational Therapy Assistants* (2nd ed.). St. Louis, MO: Elsevier Mosby, Inc. Pages 207-208, 213-214.

Wagenfeld, A & Kaldenberg, J. (2005). *Foundations of Pediatric Practice for the Occupational Therapy Assistant*. Thorofare, NJ: SLACK, Inc. Page 94.

51. Correct Answer: 2

MCP joint ulnar drift is a characteristic deformity associated with rheumatoid arthritis. To protect the MCP joints, individuals who have rheumatoid arthritis should avoid movements that place these joints in ulnar deviation.

Incorrect Answers:

1, 3, 4: Wrist extension, wrist ulnar deviation, and composite finger extension are not deforming forces inherent to the activities that seem to cause pain for this individual.

Reference: Early, M. B. (2006). *Physical Dysfunction Practice Skills for the Occupational Therapy Assistant* (2nd ed.). St. Louis, MO: Elsevier Mosby, Inc. Pages 567, 576-578.

52. Correct Answer: 4

The difference in height between the toilet and the wheelchair may cause problems with transferring. This should be assessed prior to recommending adaptive equipment or completing a manual muscle test.

Incorrect Answers:

1: A bedside commode chair would not maximize the patient's independence in toileting.

2: Individuals who have an incomplete T_2 spinal cord injury are typically able to transfer independently to a variety of surfaces without assistive devices..

3: This may be completed under the direction of the OTR, but would not be the **NEXT** action that the COTA should take.

Reference: Early, M. B. (2006). *Physical Dysfunction Practice Skills for the Occupational Therapy Assistant* (2nd ed.). St. Louis, MO: Elsevier Mosby, Inc. Pages 317-319, 545.

53. Correct Answer: 1

An individual who has Parkinson's disease has difficulty shifting weight to take steps. The safest method to turn using a walker is to stay close to the walker stand with a wide base of support and move slowly. The individual should also be taught to use a proper gait pattern to minimize fall-risk.

Incorrect Answers:

2: Turning the walker and then moving the legs could cause a fall.

3: Moving the walker to one side and reaching for support could cause the individual to loose balance.

4: Placing one hand on the counter and the other on the walker would provide an uneven base of support.

Reference: Early, M. B. (2006). *Physical Dysfunction Practice Skills for the Occupational Therapy Assistant* (2nd ed.). St. Louis, MO: Elsevier Mosby, Inc. Pages 298-299.

Sample Items

54. *Correct Answer: 2*

Blowing bubbles is a motivating play activity that promotes oral-motor movements.

Incorrect Answers:

1, 4: Liquids from an ice-pop and fruit juices are contraindicated for children who have immature oral motor control during the initial stages of treatment. Also, the cold temperature of the ice-pop would decrease oral-motor control.

3:     This task is developmentally inappropriate.

Reference: Solomon, J. W. & O'Brien, J. C. (2006). *Pediatric Skills for Occupational Therapy Assistants* (2nd ed.). St. Louis, MO: Elsevier Mosby, Inc. Page 346.

55. *Correct Answer: 1*

Carrying one small basket of clothes at a time reduces stress on the muscles of the back.

Incorrect Answers:

2:     Large bundles of wet clothes puts unnecessary stress on the back.

3, 4: Forward bending and twisting are contraindicated.

Reference: Early, M. B. (2006). *Physical Dysfunction Practice Skills for the Occupational Therapy Assistant* (2nd ed.). St. Louis, MO: Elsevier Mosby, Inc. Pages 196-197.

Pendleton, H. M. & Schultz-Krohn, W. (2006). *Pedretti's Occupational Therapy: Practice Skills for Physical Dysfunction* (6th ed.). St. Louis, MO: Elsevier Mosby, Inc. Pages 1044-1045, 1052-1053.

56. *Correct Answer: 2*

To maintain correct hip position, the affected leg must be abducted. Placing a wedge between the legs will position the hip in neutral alignment.

Incorrect Answers:

1, 3, 4: These positions do not prevent adduction or rotation of the affected hip.

Reference: Early, M. B. (2006). *Physical Dysfunction Practice Skills for the Occupational Therapy Assistant* (2nd ed.). St. Louis, MO: Elsevier Mosby, Inc. Page 621.

57. *Correct Answer: 2*

Changes in a client's performance should always be discussed with the client prior to changing any aspect of the intervention.

Incorrect Answers:

1: Unless the client signs a consent form, contacting the significant other violates the client's privacy and rights.

3: The COTA should not make changes to the intervention until talking with the client and the OTR.

4: The COTA may elect to review the treatment plan and goals with the patient after discussing observations and concerns with the client.

Reference: Early, M. B. (2006). *Physical Dysfunction Practice Skills for the Occupational Therapy Assistant* (2nd ed.). St. Louis, MO: Elsevier Mosby, Inc. Pages 70-71, 75-76.

58. *Correct Answer: 1*

These symptoms are consistent with autonomic dysreflexia which is life-threatening. The INITIAL action is to regard this as a medical emergency and call for help.

Incorrect Answers:

2: This may be a second step determined by the medical staff, but is not the most appropriate initial action.

3: The COTA and the medical team should monitor the individual closely; however, it is not the most appropriate action.

4: This is an inappropriate action which would waste time critical to the individual's medical well-being.

Reference: Early, M. B. (2006). *Physical Dysfunction Practice Skills for the Occupational Therapy Assistant* (2nd ed.). St. Louis, MO: Elsevier Mosby, Inc. Page 533.

59. *Correct Answer: 4*

All clients have the right to refuse treatment; however, to maintain therapy participation the client should be provided with an alternative choice of activity.

Incorrect Answers:

1: The cultural diversity and rights of all group participants must be acknowledged and respected.

2: The COTA may suggest that the client discuss the conflict with a pastoral counselor; however, this does not address the issue of encouraging the client to participate in therapy.

3: Exploring the conflict will not enhance task performance.

Reference: Early, M. B. (2006). *Physical Dysfunction Practice Skills for the Occupational Therapy Assistant* (2nd ed.). St. Louis, MO: Elsevier Mosby, Inc. Pages 187-188.

60. *Correct Answers: 3*

The social aspects of dining are enhanced if the resients who have hearing impairments are seated at a round table. This allows the residents to clearly see and make eye contact with others when talking.

Incorrect Answers:

1, 2, 4: Environmental noises, distractions, and glare should be minimized to enable residents who have hearing impairments participate in social conversations.

Reference: Byers-Connon, S., Lohman, H., Padilla, R. L. (2004). *Occupational Therapy with Elders: Strategies for the COTA* (2nd ed.). St. Louis, MO: Elsevier Mosby, Inc. Page 16.

61. *Correct Answer: 1*

It is **MOST IMPORTANT** to reinforce the principles of energy conservation by making sure that the supplies are available and within easy reach.

Incorrect Answers:

2, 4: Patient's who have COPD should be seated during self-care tasks. Placing a chair outside of the bathroom is not helpful.

3: Using spray deodorants and powders is contraindicated for patients who have COPD.

Reference: Byers-Connon, S., Lohman, H., Padilla, R. L. (2004). *Occupational Therapy with Elders: Strategies for the COTA* (2nd ed.). St. Louis, MO: Elsevier Mosby, Inc. Page 309.

62. Correct Answer: 1

Large print and high-contrast colors is **BEST** for enabling a client who has decreased visual acuity to use the remaining vision to enhance functional performance.

Incorrect Answers:

2: Fluorescent bulbs produce glare or shadows on work surfaces that may interfere with visual acuity.

3: Keeping items on the countertop may make these items more accessible; however, would not compensate for a visual acuity deficit.

4: Glass panels on cabinet doors may produce reflective glare which further interferes with visual acuity.

Reference: Early, M. B. (2006). *Physical Dysfunction Practice Skills for the Occupational Therapy Assistant* (2nd ed.). St. Louis, MO: Elsevier Mosby, Inc. Page 444.

63. Correct Answer: 2

Homonymous hemianopsia **TYPICALLY** results after a CVA of the posterior cerebral artery. Hemianopsia affects the visual field of both eyes and results in a neglect or inattention to a specific visual space.

Incorrect Answers:

1: A client who has figure-ground deficits has difficulty distinguishing a specific feature from the background (e.g., how many cookies are on each pan).

3: Reduced depth perception may affect a client's ability to judge distance. This would impact the ability to place a cookie tray on the oven rack, but would not affect a specific field of vision.

4: Laterality deficits impair the client's ability to distinguish between right and left sides, but do not result in avoiding one side of the environment.

Reference: Early, M. B. (2006). *Physical Dysfunction Practice Skills for the Occupational Therapy Assistant* (2nd ed.). St. Louis, MO: Elsevier Mosby, Inc. Pages 445-472.

64. Correct Answer: 2

A voice-message alarm can be programmed by a caregiver to alert a client when it is time to take a medication and which medications should be taken.

Incorrect Answers:

1, 3, 4: Use of these devices does not cue the client to take the medication at a specific time.

Reference: Byers-Connon, S., Lohman, H., Padilla, R. L. (2004). *Occupational Therapy with Elders: Strategies for the COTA* (2nd ed.). St. Louis, MO: Elsevier Mosby, Inc. Pages 171-172.

65. *Correct Answer: 2*

The **PRIMARY** goal of intervention should be for the client to learn basic personal life management skills for independent living skills and self-reliance.

Incorrect Answers:

1: Residing in a group living environment fosters dependency.

3: Engaging the client in leisure activities with friends may not support a sober/substance-free lifestyle.

4: Identifying work-related stressors does not address the client's own coping and lifestyle management strategies.

Reference: Early, M. B. (2009). *Mental Health Concepts and Techniques for the Occupational Therapy Assistant* (4th ed.). Baltimore, MD: Wolters Kluwer - Lippincott Williams & Wilkins. Pages 160-162, 529.

Cara, E. & MacRae, A. (2005). *Psychosocial Occupational Therapy* (2nd ed.). NY: Thompson Delmar, Inc. Page 592.

66. *Correct Answer: 4*

Decreased platelet level can result in an increased risk of prolonged bleeding if the patient is cut. Activities requiring sharp tools present a risk management issue and are **CONTRAINDICATED**.

Incorrect Answers:

1, 2, 3: There are no special precautions with these materials that need to be considered for patients who have this condition.

Reference: Early, M. B. (2006). *Physical Dysfunction Practice Skills for the Occupational Therapy Assistant* (2nd ed.). St. Louis, MO: Elsevier Mosby, Inc. Page 679.

67. *Correct Answer: 1*

Collaborating with the participants to select an activity that is valuable and meaningful is BEST for enhancing task-specific performance.

Incorrect Answers:

2, 3, 4: These options are not client-centered and may not promote maximal participation toward the stated goal.

Reference: Early, M. B. (2009). *Mental Health Concepts and Techniques for the Occupational Therapy Assistant* (4th ed.). Baltimore, MD: Wolters Kluwer - Lippincott Williams & Wilkins. Pages 170-171.

68. *Correct Answer: 3*

This activity is **BEST** because the COTA can determine the impact of the client's condition on an activity that is meaningful and important to the client.

Incorrect Answers:

1, 2: The task that is important to the client is playing the piano. These choices may improve strength and fine motor control, but do not incorporate the client's valued activity.

4:    Actually engaging in a preferred activity is more beneficial than passive participation.

Reference: Early, M. B. (2006). *Physical Dysfunction Practice Skills for the Occupational Therapy Assistant* (2nd ed.). St. Louis, MO: Elsevier Mosby, Inc. Page 360.

69. Correct Answer: 2

During a parallel task group, individuals work in the presence of other participants, but social interaction is not necessary. Since the patient is just beginning to tolerate being in the presence of others, this is the **BEST** initial activity for this patient.

Incorrect Answers:

1, 3, 4: Values clarification, team sports, and community outing groups require direct involvement with other individuals and would be overwhelming to the patient based on the patient's current status.

Reference: Early, M. B. (2009). *Mental Health Concepts and Techniques for the Occupational Therapy Assistant* (4ᵗʰ ed.). Baltimore, MD: Wolters Kluwer - Lippincott Williams & Wilkins. Pages 165, 347.

70. Correct Answer: 1

Learning energy conservation techniques during the **INITIAL** phase of rehabilitation will promote the client's functional performance within the limitations of the disorder.

Incorrect Answers:

2, 3, 4: These options may be considered later in the intervention process based on the client's needs.

Reference: Early, M. B. (2006). *Physical Dysfunction Practice Skills for the Occupational Therapy Assistant* (2ⁿᵈ ed.). St. Louis, MO: Elsevier Mosby, Inc. Page 675.

71. Correct Answer: 1

This activity is **BEST** for promoting bilateral use of the upper extremities at a developmentally appropriate level.

Incorrect Answers:

2, 3, 4: These are play activities for typically developing children between the ages of 4 and 8 years of age.

Reference: Solomon, J. W. & O'Brien, J. C. (2006). *Pediatric Skills for Occupational Therapy Assistants* (2ⁿᵈ ed.). St. Louis, MO: Elsevier Mosby, Inc. Pages 124-125, 463-464.

72. Correct Answer: 2

Activities are considered therapeutic when they have inherent value to the patient and relate to the patient's needs and goals. **INITIAL** activities for inpatients who have major depression should guarantee success.

Incorrect Answers:

1: Completing a simple project may not have inherent value for the patients.

3: These areas would not be the **INITIAL** focus of a group of inpatients who have major depression.

4: Using OT as a diversion is an inappropriate use of services.

Reference: Early, M. B. (2009). *Mental Health Concepts and Techniques for the Occupational Therapy Assistant* (4ᵗʰ ed.). Baltimore, MD: Wolters Kluwer - Lippincott Williams & Wilkins. Page 295.

73. Correct Answer: 2

This choice is an inhibitory technique and is therefore **MOST EFFECTIVE** for reducing muscle tone and arousal state.

Incorrect Answers:

1, 3, 4: These are facilitation techniques used to increase muscle tone.

Reference: Solomon, J. W. & O'Brien, J. C. (2006). *Pediatric Skills for Occupational Therapy Assistants* (2nd ed.). St. Louis, MO: Elsevier Mosby, Inc. Page 231.

74. Correct Answer: 1

This is the **BEST** choice as it is the only one that requires bilateral hand-use.

Incorrect Answers:

2, 3, 4: These answers are most often performed unilaterally. Therefore, they are not the **BEST** activities for promoting bilateral hand-use.

Reference: Solomon, J. W. & O'Brien, J. C. (2006). *Pediatric Skills for Occupational Therapy Assistants* (2nd ed.). St. Louis, MO: Elsevier Mosby, Inc. Pages 463-464.

Case-Smith, J. (2001). *Occupational Therapy for Children* (4th ed.). St. Louis, MO: Mosby, Inc. Pages 321-322.

75. Correct Answer: 2

Environmental adaptations that are simple and familiar to the individual are **MOST BENEFICIAL** for decreasing confusion and fostering independence.

Incorrect Answers:

1: Painting the walls may cause increased stimulation and the individual may not be able to process information.

3: Dim lighting would decrease the individual's ability to locate visual cues and may also increase fall-risks.

4: Multi-sensory cues may lead to increased confusion and agitation that may promote wandering.

Reference: Early, M. B. (2009). *Mental Health Concepts and Techniques for the Occupational Therapy Assistant* (4th ed.). Baltimore, MD: Wolters Kluwer - Lippincott Williams & Wilkins. Pages 314-315.

76. Correct Answer: 1

Using this breathing technique during exertion is **MOST EFFECTIVE** for reducing demands on the lungs and cardiovascular system.

Incorrect Answers:

2, 3, 4: These techniques are not effective for managing the symptoms of COPD.

Reference: Early, M. B. (2006). *Physical Dysfunction Practice Skills for the Occupational Therapy Assistant* (2nd ed.). St. Louis, MO: Elsevier Mosby, Inc. Pages 671-672.

Radomski, M.V. & Trombly-Latham, C. A. (2008). *Occupational Therapy for Physical Dysfunction* (6th ed.). Baltimore, MD: Wolters Kluwer -Lippincott Williams & Wilkins. Pages 1309-1310.

77. Correct Answer: 1

This activity encourages fine-motor control and isolated finger movement to improve pencil grasp development.

Incorrect Answers:

2, 3, 4: These activities do not provide an effective means for improving fine-motor or isolated finger movement patterns to assist appropriate pencil grasp development.

Reference: Case-Smith, J. (2001). *Occupational Therapy for Children* (4th ed.). St. Louis, MO: Mosby, Inc. Page 547.

78. Correct Answer: 1

Creating rhymes about school assignments is **MOST BENEFICIAL** for helping the student to process, remember, and recall information through the use of language cues.

Incorrect Answers:

2, 3, 4: There is no evidence that these activities are beneficial for promoting long-term visual memory storage.

Reference: Case-Smith, J. (2005). *Occupational Therapy for Children* (5th ed.). St. Louis, MO: Mosby, Inc. Page 436.

Wagenfeld, A & Kaldenberg, J. (2005). *Foundations of Pediatric Practice for the Occupational Therapy Assistant*. Thorofare, NJ: SLACK, Inc. Page 223.

79. Correct Answer: 4

This child must **INITIALLY** learn to integrate and process sensory input as a precursor to learning Braille.

Incorrect Answers:

1: This option is contraindicated as an initial intervention for tactile defensiveness.
2, 3: These options do not address sensory processing deficits related to tactile defensiveness.

Reference: Solomon, J. W. & O'Brien, J. C. (2006). *Pediatric Skills for Occupational Therapy Assistants* (2nd ed.). St. Louis, MO: Elsevier Mosby, Inc. Pages 282-283.

80. Correct Answer: 2

Intense pain or an unpleasant experience may cause a temporary vasovagal response by the autonomic nervous system. As a result the heart rate and blood drop, which reduces the blood flow to the brain. This results in a feeling of warmth, lightheadedness, dimming vision and hearing, and even fainting (vasovagal syncope). The client must be quickly reclined with the legs elevated in order for blood pressure to return to normal.

Incorrect Answers:

1, 4: This will not assist with elevating the client's blood pressure.
3: This is likely to further contribute to the client's lowering blood pressure.

Reference: Early, M.B. (2006). *Physical Dysfunction: Practice Skills for the Occupational Therapy Assistant* (2nd ed.). St. Louis, MO: Elsevier Mosby, Inc. Page 55.

81. *Correct Answer: 3*

Directing the light source from behind the client's shoulder will prevent the glare source from directing towards the client's eyes while reading the magazine.

Incorrect Answers:

1, 2: These do not address the client's preferred leisure activity of reading a favorite magazine.

4:   The magazine may not be available in matte finish, therefore this option may not assist the client in continuing to read their favorite magazine

Reference: Byers-Connon, S., Lohman, H, & Padilla, R.L. (eds.) (2004). *Occupational Therapy with Elders* (2nd ed.). St Louis, MO: Elsevier Mosby, Inc. Page 207.

82. *Correct answer: 1*

Homemaking environments, habits, and routines vary from culture to culture. It is therefore important for the COTA to recognize this client's culture and values when assisting them towards their goals.

Incorrect Answers:

2, 4: These do not take into account the client's established homemaking habits and routines.

3:   The COTA needs to first establish if this activity respects the client's culture and values before incorporating it into a treatment session.

Reference: Early, M.B. (2009). *Mental Health Concepts and Techniques for the Occupational Therapy Assistant* (4th Ed.). Baltimore, MD: Wolters Kluwer-Lippincott. Williams & Wilkins. Pages 244, 500.

83. *Correct Answer: 3*

To qualify for Medicare reimbursement, the documented OT treatment plan **MUST** include long-term functional goals that are deemed medically necessary.

Incorrect Answers:

1, 2, 4: Documentation of these is not required to meet Medicare requirements for reimbursement.

Reference: Byers-Connon, S., Lohman, H., Padilla, R.L. (2004). *Occupational Therapy with Elders: Strategies for the COTA* (2nd ed.). St. Louis, MO: Elsevier Mosby, Inc. Pages 380-383, 390.

Borcherding, S. (2005). *Documentation Manual for Writing SOAP Notes in Occupational Therapy* (2nd ed.). Thorofare, NJ: SLACK, Inc. Pages 40-41.

84. Correct Answer: 1

The "A" section of the SOAP note should reflect an assessment of the situation in relation to the established goal(s). In this case the assessment is reflected **BEST** in option 1.

Incorrect Answers:

2: The patient is already independent in upper extremity dressing with minimal assistance. It is unlikely that the patient will require assistance for most self-care at discharge.

3: This is subjective information and does not need to be reflected in a progress note.

4: Although it is not known from the information presented if the patient is independent in upper extremity dressing when seated in a wheelchair, this information is best to include in the "O" section of an SOAP note.

Reference: Early, M. B. (2006). *Physical Dysfunction Practice Skills for the Occupational Therapy Assistant* (2nd ed.). St. Louis, MO: Elsevier Mosby, Inc. Page 87.

Borcherding, S. (2005). *Documentation Manual for Writing SOAP Notes in Occupational Therapy* (2nd ed.). Thorofare, NJ: SLACK, Inc. Pages 164-167, 226-227.

85. Correct Answer: 3

Rubber-sole shoes will help the elder obtain more secure footing and minimize the risk of falling.

Incorrect Answers:

1, 2: Using a walker and caregiver assistance when it is not necessary, promotes dependence.

4: Walking with a shuffle gait promotes abnormal gait patterns and does not reduce the fall risk.

Reference: Byers-Connon, S., Lohman, H., Padilla, R. L. (2004). *Occupational Therapy with Elders: Strategies for the COTA* (2nd ed.). St. Louis, MO: Elsevier Mosby, Inc. Page 189.

86. Correct Answer: 1

The COTA should **INITIALLY** collaborate with the client to determine the barriers to participation in OT and the potential solutions.

Incorrect Answers:

2, 4: An independent home program and monthly re-evaluations are less effective than active participation in OT at this stage of the client's rehabilitation.

3: A home health agency may be indicated if the client is "home bound" and qualified by nursing, PT, or speech to receive OT services.

Reference: Crepeau, E.B., Cohn, E.S. & Schell, B.A.B. (2009). *Willard & Spackman's Occupational Therapy* (11th ed.). Philadelphia, PA: Lippincott Williams & Wilkins. Page 956.

Early, M.B. (2006). *Physical Dysfunction Practice Skills for the Occupational Therapy Assistant* (2nd ed.). St. Louis, MO: Elsevier Mosby, Inc. Pages 64, 72.

87. *Correct Answer: 3*

The discharge summary is a key document used when assessing outcomes. It must contain objective information about functional progress from initiation of OT to discharge.

Incorrect Answers:

1, 2, 4: This information is useful, but is not required in a discharge summary or when assessing outcomes.

Reference: Early, M. B. (2006). *Physical Dysfunction Practice Skills for the Occupational Therapy Assistant* (2nd ed.). St. Louis, MO: Elsevier Mosby, Inc. Pages 91, 100, 137.

88. *Correct Answer: 4*

In an acute-care setting, treatment emphasis is on improving self-care skills for patients who have major depression. Progress toward goals in this area need to be included in the discharge summary for reimbursement purposes as well as future intervention planning.

Incorrect Answers:

1: Specific job-performance skills are not addressed in an acute-care facility.

2: Gross and fine motor skills alone typically are not addressed in an acute psychiatric setting

3: Scores from a single test do not provide information about outcomes

Reference: Early, M. B. (2006). *Physical Dysfunction Practice Skills for the Occupational Therapy Assistant* (2nd ed.). St. Louis, MO: Elsevier Mosby, Inc. Pages 91, 100, 137.

Early, M. B. (2000). *Mental Health Concepts and Techniques for the Occupational Therapy Assistant* (3rd ed.). Baltimore, MD: Lippincott Williams & Wilkins. Pages 477-478.

89. *Correct Answer: 2*

The purpose of a wellness program is to promote health and minimize the impact of pre-existing disease on occupational role performance.

Incorrect Answers:

1: This does not provide guidance about implementing lifestyle changes.

3: It is not the role of the COTA to recommend over-the-counter medications.

4: Individual sessions, if needed, may be recommended at the completion of the program or if a client is experiencing difficulty.

Reference: Byers-Connon, S., Lohman, H., Padilla, R. L. (2004). *Occupational Therapy with Elders: Strategies for the COTA* (2nd ed.). St. Louis, MO: Elsevier Mosby, Inc. Page 58.

90. *Correct Answer: 1*

A COTA requires close supervision at entry-level, requiring daily, direct contact.

Incorrect Answers:

2: Service competence must be reassessed at the new place of employment.

3: This may be used as a part of service competence; but is not the initial step.

4: Review of documentation does not provide adequate supervision.

Reference: Pendleton, H. M. & Schultz-Krohn, W. (2006). *Pedretti's Occupational Therapy: Practice Skills for Physical Dysfunction* (6th ed.). St. Louis, MO: Elsevier Mosby, Inc. Pages 942-943.

91. *Correct Answer: 4*

Administering a developmental skills checklist after establishing service competency, is a typical responsibility of a COTA. This task does not require interpretation beyond the scope of practice for a newly certified COTA.

Incorrect Answers:

1:     A sensory integration assessment requires advanced training and is typically administered and scored by an OTR.

2, 3: These duties are the responsibility of an OTR.

Reference: Solomon, J. W. & O'Brien, J. C. (2006). *Pediatric Skills for Occupational Therapy Assistants* (2nd ed.). St. Louis, MO: Elsevier Mosby, Inc. Pages 153-154.

92. *Correct Answer: 1*

The use of occupational therapy aides must be done in accordance with specific state practice acts and governing laws.

Incorrect Answers:

2:     It is not essential for the COTA to be familiar with specific critical demands listed on the aide's job description.

3, 4: These are not essential to know prior to assigning tasks to the aide.

Reference: Pendleton, H. M. & Schultz-Krohn, W. (2006). *Pedretti's Occupational Therapy: Practice Skills for Physical Dysfunction* (6th ed.). St. Louis, MO: Elsevier Mosby, Inc. Page 947.

93. *Correct answer: 2*

The "O" section of a SOAP note is the objective part of the note that should contain measurable and observable data.

Incorrect Answers:

1: This is part of the plan that is included in the "P" section of a SOAP note.

3: This is subjective information that is included in the "S" section of a SOAP note.

4: This is assessment information that is included in the "A" section of a SOAP note.

Reference: Early, M. B. (2006). *Physical Dysfunction Practice Skills for the Occupational Therapy Assistant* (2nd ed.). St. Louis, MO: Elsevier Mosby, Inc. Page 87.

Borcherding, S. (2005). *Documentation Manual for Writing SOAP Notes in Occupational Therapy* (2nd ed.). Thorofare, NJ: SLACK, Inc. Pages 53-54.

94. *Correct Answer: 2*

Progress notes should provide evidence about the client's progress in relation to the established functional goals.

Incorrect Answers:

1, 4: Subjective progress and progress related to other patients is not needed.

3:    Anticipated functional outcomes are subjective and not evidence-based.

Reference: Early, M. B. (2006). *Physical Dysfunction Practice Skills for the Occupational Therapy Assistant* (2ⁿᵈ ed.). St. Louis, MO: Elsevier Mosby, Inc. Page 100.

95. *Correct Answer: 1*

Patients at this level should be monitored at all times. To ensure safety, all equipment and supplies must be returned to a storage area as per facility policy.

Incorrect Answers:

2, 3, 4: These are procedural routines that may vary depending on the group and the facility.

Reference: Early, M. B. (2009). *Mental Health Concepts and Techniques for the Occupational Therapy Assistant* (4ᵗʰ ed.). Baltimore, MD: Wolters Kluwer - Lippincott Williams & Wilkins. Page 328.

96. *Correct Answer: 3*

To minimize infection risk, the client should use a personally-owned shaver. Using an electric razor decreases the risk of cuts and is easier to use with the non-dominant hand.

Incorrect Answers:

1: A straight-edge razor increases risk of injury. Alcohol is not a universal germicide.

2: To minimize the risk of infection/cross contamination, personal hygiene items should not be shared.

4: Disposable straight-edge razors may be difficult for the client to use with the non-dominant extremity.

Reference: Early, M. B. (2006). *Physical Dysfunction Practice Skills for the Occupational Therapy Assistant* (2ⁿᵈ ed.). St. Louis, MO: Elsevier Mosby, Inc. Pages 254, 49-51.

97. *Correct Answer: 3*

Reimbursement from Medicare is determined by the number of "therapy minutes" that are documented in the minimum data set (MDS).

Incorrect Answers:

1, 2, 4: This information is not a requirement of the Medicare Prospective Payment System.

Reference: Byers-Connon, S., Lohman, H., Padilla, R. L. (2004). *Occupational Therapy with Elders: Strategies for the COTA* (2ⁿᵈ ed.). St. Louis, MO: Elsevier Mosby, Inc. Page 67.

98. *Correct Answer: 2*

   Supervision and structured learning provide an effective means for establishing service competency with splinting.

   Incorrect Answers:

   1, 4: Use of visual aids from textbooks, reviewing class notes, or reading journal articles does not meet the requirement for establishing service competency in actually fabricating a splint.

   3:    Making a check list of key tips for splinting may serve as a helpful reminder, but does not ensure service competency for fabricating splints.

   Reference: Crepeau, E. B., Cohn, E. S. & Schell, B. A. B. (2009). *Willard & Spackman's Occupational Therapy* (11th ed.). Philadelphia, PA: Lippincott Williams & Wilkins. Pages 943.

   Solomon, J. W. & O'Brien, J. C. (2006). *Pediatric Skills for Occupational Therapy Assistants* (2nd ed.). St. Louis, MO: Elsevier Mosby, Inc. Pages 13-14.

99. *Correct Answer: 2*

   An interactive discussion is not only informative, but can be tailored to the participants' interests and concerns.

   Incorrect Answers:

   1:    The topic is to address disease process management, not assessment. Public members are usually more interested in how problems will be addressed; this method is more appropriate for an audience of healthcare team members.

   3, 4: Providing a simulation of a therapy session or demonstrating an exercise program does not provide a broad perspective about the services that OT has to offer for individuals who have this disease. Additionally, these do not address the specific concerns of the attendees.

   Reference: Early, M. B. (2006). *Physical Dysfunction Practice Skills for the Occupational Therapy Assistant* (2nd ed.). St. Louis, MO: Elsevier Mosby, Inc. Pages 187-189, 568.

100.   *Correct Answer: 1*

   The most effective method of communicating the value of OT services to this audience is to use an outcomes measure. This will provide parents with objective information about the positive impact of a student's skills and abilities on employability.

   Incorrect Answers:

   2, 3, 4: Describing disability statistics, demonstrating assistive technology, and outlining parental responsibility do not reflect the outcome of OT intervention, which is improved occupational performance.

   Reference: Early, M. B. (2009). *Mental Health Concepts and Techniques for the Occupational Therapy Assistant* (4th ed.). Baltimore, MD: Wolters Kluwer - Lippincott Williams & Wilkins. Pages 383-384, 516.

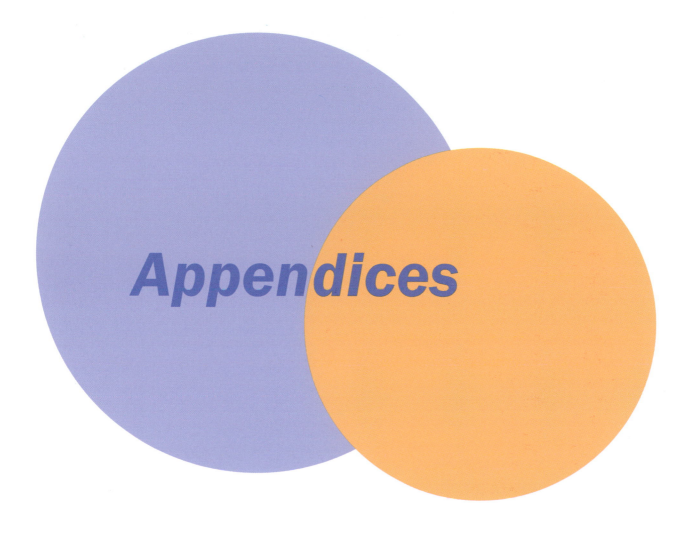

Appendices

Certification Examination Readiness Tool

for the

CERTIFIED OCCUPATIONAL THERAPY ASSISTANT COTA®

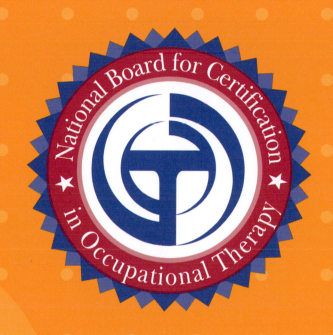

A Publication of the
National Board for Certification in Occupational Therapy, Inc.

"This tool really helped me identify my strengths and weaknesses. After using this I developed a structured study plan."

- NBCOT® Exam Candidate

"I used this tool as a part of a class assignment before the students went out on Level II fieldwork. The tool helped to formulate fieldwork goals and objectives."

- Academic Fieldwork Coordinator

"Doing this calmed my nerves... I realized that I had covered most of these skills already. It gave me confidence to continue with my exam preparation."

- NBCOT Exam Candidate

National Board for Certification in Occupational Therapy, Inc.
12 South Summit Avenue, Suite 100
Gaithersburg, MD 20877-4150
http://www.nbcot.org

This tool contains the validated domains, tasks, and skills resulting from the 2007 NBCOT® practice analysis study. **The tool is designed for candidates planning to take the NBCOT CERTIFIED OCCUPATIONAL THERAPY ASSISTANT COTA® examination January 2009 onwards.** It is one of several official NBCOT examination preparation tools - including study guides and online practice tests - developed to assist COTA exam candidates with their test preparation.

In line with certification industry standards, the foundation of the NBCOT certification examinations is based on a practice analysis study. NBCOT periodically conducts practice analysis studies as a basis for developing, maintaining, and defending the content validity of its certification examinations. The last practice analysis study – conducted by NBCOT in 2007 – identified the domains and tasks performed by COTA practitioners, along with the knowledge and skill required to perform them. Results from the study were used to construct the COTA examination test blueprint that will guide examination development for the NBCOT COTA certification examinations beginning January 2009.

About This Tool

This tool lists the validated domains, tasks, and skill statements used to guide examination development for the COTA certification examinations beginning January 2009.

To the right of the skill statements, there is a series of columns and corresponding checkboxes, titled:

I have performed skill independently

I have performed skill under supervision

I have observed other practitioners performing skill

I have no experience with skill

How To Use This Tool

This tool can be used in two ways to help assess readiness for the certification examination:

1. To review the validated domains, tasks and skill statements used by NBCOT item writers during the examination item development process:

    - Example of how a COTA exam item is developed:

    Domain: 01 Gather information and formulate conclusions regarding the client's needs priorities to develop a client-centered intervention plan

    Task: 01.02 Contribute comprehensive information regarding the impact of current condition(s) and context(s) on the client's occupational performance in order to assist the OTR in formulating an intervention plan.

    Skill: c)   Identifying activities to enhance the client's occupational performance

    Exam Item: A COTA is planning intervention for a 5-year-old child who has moderate autism. Which environment is MOST BENEFICIAL for promoting the child's play skills?

    A)   In a clinic that has a variety of brightly colored mechanical toys

    B)   At a familiar location with several developmentally-appropriate toys*

    C)   In a secluded area with multiple age-appropriate games and action toys

    D)   During a group activity that fosters sensory stimulation and free play opportunities

2. As a self-evaluation tool, the user may choose to indicate their level of experience for each skill by marking the corresponding checkbox.

Example of self-evaluation:

Skill	Performed independently	Under supervision	Observed others	No experience
01.04 Provide information to the OTR regarding the need for referral to other professionals or services in order to facilitate comprehensive, quality care.				
a. Communicating with other team members and community organizations	√			
b. Recognizing the parameters of other service delivery models (e.g. criteria, least restrictive environment, acuity)		√		

Disclaimer: Using this tool cannot guarantee your success on the NBCOT® certification examination. However, candidates may consider using the tool to guide their test preparation strategies or as a basis for discussion with their program director or fieldwork educator.

01 GATHER INFORMATION AND FORMULATE CONCLUSIONS REGARDING THE CLIENT'S NEEDS AND PRIORITIES TO DEVELOP A CLIENT-CENTERED INTERVENTION PLAN

Skill	Performed independently	Under supervision	Observed others	No experience
01.01 Gather information on an ongoing basis using appropriate tools, procedures, and protocols in order to identify factors that impact participation in occupation.				
a. Conducting oneself in a therapeutic manner to gather essential data				
b. Gathering client history related to engagement in occupations				
c. Administering assessments in accordance with protocols				
d. Identifying client needs, problems, concerns, and priorities about occupations and daily life activity performance				
e. Identifying factors that support or hinder occupational performance				
f. Recognizing and responding to unexpected client responses while gathering information				
01.02 Contribute comprehensive information regarding the impact of current condition(s) and context(s) on the client's occupational performance in order to assist the OTR in formulating an intervention plan.				
a. Identifying appropriate frames of reference and models of practice				
b. Analyzing activities for the selection of occupation-based interventions consistent with client roles, habits, routines, and current abilities				
c. Identifying activities to enhance the client's occupational performance				
d. Determining factors that impact occupational performance				
e. Interpreting the importance of contextual factors that impact engagement in occupation				
01.03 Collaborate with the OTR, client, and relevant others using a team approach in order to prioritize client centered goals throughout the continuum of care, guided by evidence and the principles of best practice.				
a. Identifying the client's priorities and desired outcomes				
b. Identifying the need to continue, modify, or discontinue services based on the client's responses to intervention				
c. Communicating with the client and team members about client goals and outcomes				
d. Determining frequency and duration of intervention based on expected outcomes				
e. Following discharge and transition planning procedures				
01.04 Provide information to the OTR regarding the need for referral to other professionals or services in order to facilitate comprehensive, quality care.				
a. Communicating with other team members and community organizations				
b. Recognizing the parameters of other service delivery models (e.g. criteria, least restrictive environment, acuity)				

Appendices

A

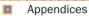

Skill	Performed independently	Under supervision	Observed others	No experience
02.01 Implement the treatment plan by using critical reasoning to select interventions and approaches consistent with general medical, neurological, and musculoskeletal conditions and client needs in order to achieve functional outcomes within areas of occupation.				
a. Conducting oneself in a therapeutic manner to facilitate change based on a client's general medical, neurological, and/or musculoskeletal condition				
b. Selecting and implementing compensatory, remedial, biomechanical, and/or preventive interventions as related to general medical, neurological, and/or musculoskeletal conditions				
c. Facilitating individual and group occupation-based activities consistent with a client's general medical, neurological, and/or musculoskeletal condition and current abilities				
d. Using facilitation and handling principles and techniques consistent with general medical, neurological, and/or musculoskeletal condition				
e. Adhering to protocols for applying physical agent modalities				
f. Selecting, designing, fabricating, and/or modifying common splints based on general medical, neurological, and/or musculoskeletal conditions and client needs				
g. Selecting, designing, fabricating and/or modifying adaptive equipment or assistive devices based on medical, neurological, and/or musculoskeletal conditions and client needs				
h. Adhering to protocols for implementing interventions for facilitating chewing and swallowing specific to general medical conditions.				
i. Teaching positioning and physical transfer techniques consistent with activity demands, client abilities				
j. Using neurobehavioral techniques for skill development				
02.02 Implement the treatment plan by using critical reasoning to select interventions and approaches consistent with developmental level, pediatric conditions, and/or congenital anomalies and client needs in order to achieve functional outcomes within areas of occupation.				
a. Using occupation in a therapeutic manner to promote function based on a client's roles, habits and routines, and developmental abilities				
b. Conducting oneself in a therapeutic manner to facilitate change consistent with developmental needs				
c. Selecting and implementing interventions consistent with developmental level, pediatric conditions and/or congenital anomalies				

Skill	Performed independently	Under supervision	Observed others	No experience
d. Using developmentally based methods and techniques to facilitate group activities				
e. Using facilitation and handling techniques during interventions consistent with developmental level, pediatric conditions, and/or congenital anomalies				
f. Using sensory integrative interventions and sensory modulation techniques				
g. Selecting, designing, fabricating, and/or modifying common splints based on developmental level, pediatric conditions, and/or congenital anomalies and client needs				
h. Selecting, designing, fabricating and/or modifying adaptive equipment or assistive devices based on developmental level, pediatric conditions, and/or congenital anomalies and client needs				
i. Adhering to protocols for implementing interventions for facilitate chewing and swallowing specific to developmental level, pediatric conditions, and/or congenital anomalies				
j. Teaching positioning and physical transfer techniques consistent with developmental level and activity demands				
k. Using neurobehavioral techniques for skill acquisition consistent with developmental level, pediatric conditions, and/or congenital anomalies				
l. Using prevocational and vocational exploration processes and procedures				
02.03 Implement the treatment plan by using critical reasoning to select interventions and approaches consistent with psychosocial and cognitive abilities, and client needs in order to achieve functional outcomes within areas of occupation.				
a. Using occupation in a therapeutic manner appropriate to psychosocial and/or cognitive abilities, client roles, habits and routines				
b. Implementing therapeutic interventions appropriate to psychosocial and/or cognitive abilities, client roles, habits and routines				
c. Conducting oneself in a therapeutic manner to facilitate change based on psychosocial and/or cognitive abilities				
d. Using compensatory, remedial, and/or preventive techniques consistent with psychosocial and/or cognitive abilities, client roles, habits and routines				
e. Selecting, designing, fabricating and/or modifying adaptive equipment or assistive devices based on psychosocial and/or cognitive abilities				
f. Planning and facilitating group activities consistent with psychosocial and/or cognitive models of practice				
g. Responding in a therapeutic manner to the needs of a client or caregiver during psychosocial interventions				

Appendices

A

Skill	Performed independently	Under supervision	Observed others	No experience
02.04 **Maximize accessibility to and mobility within a client's contexts by recommending environmental modifications in order to optimize occupational performance and/or enhance quality of life.**				
a. Identifying accessibility and risk factors				
b. Identifying and resolving mobility, seating, assistive technology, and durable medical equipment needs				
c. Making basic environmental modifications				
d. Educating the client and relevant others about the safe and effective use of environmental modifications, seating and mobility devices, durable medical equipment, and assistive technology				
02.05 **Modify intervention methods and techniques based on the client's needs and responses in order to promote occupational performance.**				
a. Identifying the need to adjust intervention techniques, adapt the environment, and/or grade the intervention activity				
b. Adjusting the intervention technique in response to variances in anticipated outcomes				
c. Adapting the environment to support participation during the intervention				
d. Grading the intervention activity based on expected progress and/or unexpected physical responses				
e. Responding appropriately to unexpected occurrences during intervention				
02.06 **Apply the principles of health promotion, wellness, prevention, and/or educational programming based on client and community needs in order to serve as a resource for occupation based program activities.**				
a. Contributing information to identify the service needs for various populations				
b. Advocating for services and resources for various populations				
c. Conducting individual and group health promotion and wellness program activities				
d. Collaborating with community based agencies				

Skill	Performed independently	Under supervision	Observed others	No experience
03.01 Maintaining ongoing competence by participating in professional development activities in order to provide effective services and promote quality care.				
a. Creating an appropriate professional development plan				
b. Engaging in professional development activities				
c. Adapting to change in the OT scope of practice				
d. Applying professional literature to the improvement of practice				
e. Determining service competency needs with guidance of the OTR				
03.02 Upholding professional standards by participating in continuous quality improvement activities and complying with safety regulations, laws, ethical codes, facility policies and procedures, and guidelines governing OT practice in order to protect the public interest				
a. Complying with federal, stage, and other types of regulatory laws and rules				
b. Identifying policies and procedures that are specific to agencies				
c. Implementing safety and risk management techniques during intervention				
d. Incorporating federally mandated guidelines into intervention plans				
e. Designing and implementing safeguards in an environment to promote safety				
f. Organizing time and services				
03.03 Document occupational therapy services using established guidelines in order to verify accountability and to meet the requirements of practice settings, accrediting bodies, regulatory agencies, and/or funding sources.				
a. Organizing documentation accurately and in accordance with practice settings, regulatory agencies, or funding sources				
b. Differentiating among financial systems for reimbursement purposes				
c. Communicating effectively through documentation				
d. Adhering to applicable regulations and guidelines related to documentation				

Appendices

A

Skill	Performed independently	Under supervision	Observed others	No experience
03.04 Articulate how occupational therapy contributes to beneficial outcomes for clients and relevant others based on evidence in order to promote quality care.				
a. Clarifying the role, responsibilities and scope of practice for OT practitioners.				
b. Developing and disseminating information about OT services				
03.05 Supervise occupational therapy students, paraprofessionals, and volunteers in accordance with professional guidelines and applicable regulations in order to support the delivery of appropriate occupational therapy services.				
a. Delegating tasks and responsibilities to supervisees as appropriate				
b. Communicating and collaborating effectively with supervisees				
c. Assessing the competence of supervisees				
d. Incorporating competency-based learning activities				
e. Developing remedial plans				

Appendices

A

National Board for Certification in Occupational Therapy, Inc.
12 South Summit Avenue, Suite 100
Gaithersburg, MD 20877-4150
P: 301.990.7979   F: 301-869.8492
www.nbcot.org

*Barnhart, P.A. (1997). *The Guide to National Professional Certification Programs (2ⁿᵈ ed.)*. Amherst, MA: HRD Press.

*Brookfield, S. (1987). *Developing Critical Thinkers*. San Francisco, CA: Jossey-Bass, Inc.

Borcherding, S. & Morreale, M. (2005). *The OTA's Guide to Writing SOAP Notes (2ⁿᵈ ed.)*. Thorofare, NJ: SLACK, Inc.

Bruce, M. & Borg, B. (2002). *Psychosocial Frames of Reference: Core for Occupation-based Practice (3ʳᵈ ed.)*. Thorofare, NJ: SLACK, Inc.

Byers-Connon, S., Lohman, H, & Padilla, RL (eds). (2004). *Occupational Therapy with Elders: Strategies for the COTA (2ⁿᵈ ed.)*. St. Louis, MO: Elsevier Mosby, Inc.

Cara, E, & MacRae, A. (2005). *Psychosocial Occupational Therapy: A Clinical Practice (2ⁿᵈ ed.)*. NY: Thomson Delmar.

Case-Smith, J. (2005). *Occupational Therapy for Children (5ᵗʰ ed.)*. St. Louis, MO: Elsevier Mosby, Inc.

Cole, M.B. (2005). *Group Dynamics in Occupational Therapy: The Theoretical Basis and Practice Application of Group Intervention (3ʳᵈ ed.)*. Thorofare, NJ: SLACK, Inc.

Coppard, B.M. & Lohman, H. (2008). *Introduction to Splinting: A Clinical-Reasoning & Problem Solving Approach (3ʳᵈ ed.)*. St. Louis, MO: Elsevier Mosby, Inc.

*Covey, S.R. (1989). *The 7 Habits of Highly Effective People*. New York: Simon & Schuster.

Crepeau, E.B., Cohn, E.S. & Schell, B.A.B. (2009). *Willard & Spackman's Occupational Therapy (11ᵗʰ ed.)*. Baltimore, MD: Wolters Kluwer - Lippincott, Williams & Wilkins.

Davis, C.M. (2006). *Patient Practitioner Interaction: An Experiential Manual for Developing the Art of Health Care (4ᵗʰ ed.)*. Thorofare, NJ: SLACK, Inc.

Early, M.B. (2009). *Mental Health Concepts and Techniques for the Occupational Therapy Assistant (4ᵗʰ ed.)*. Baltimore, MD: Wolters Kluwer -Lippincott. Williams & Wilkins.

Early, M.B. (2006). *Physical Dysfunction: Practice Skills for the Occupational Therapy Assistant (2ⁿᵈ ed.)*. St. Louis, MO: Elsevier Mosby, Inc.

*McClain, N., Richardson, B., & Wyatt, J. (2004, May-June). A profile of certification for pediatric nurses. *Pediatric Nursing*, 207-211.

McCormack, G., Jaffe, E.G. & Goodman-Lavey, M. (eds). (2003). *The Occupational Therapy Manager (4ᵗʰ ed.)*. Rockville, MD: AOTA Press.

*Microsoft (2003). Microsoft certifications benefits of certification. Retrieved from *www.microsoft.com/traincert.*

Appendices

B

Pedretti, W. & Early, M. (2006). *Pedretti's Occupational Therapy: Practice Skills for Physical Dysfunction (6th ed.).* St. Louis, MO: Elsevier Mosby, Inc.

Purtillo, R. (2005). *Ethical Dimensions in the Health Professions (4th ed.).* Philadelphia, PA: Elsevier Saunders.

Radomski, M.V. & Trombly-Latham, C. (2008). *Occupational Therapy for Physical Dysfunction (6th ed.).* Baltimore, MD: Lippincott, Williams and Wilkins.

Sames, K. (2005). *Documenting Occupational Therapy Practice.* New Jersey: Pearson Prentice Hall.

Scaffa, M. (2005). *Occupational Therapy in Community-based Practice Settings.* Philadelphia, PA: FA Davis.

Scheiman, M., Scheiman, M. & Whittaker, S. (2007). *Low Vision Rehabilitation: A Practical Guide for Occupational Therapists.* Thorofare, NJ: SLACK, Inc.

Sladyk, K, & Ryan, S. (2005). *Occupational Therapy Assistant: Principles- Practice Issues and Technology (4th ed.).* Thorofare, NJ: SLACK, Inc.

Solomon, J. & O'Brien, J. (2006). *Pediatric Skills for Occupational Therapy Assistants (2nd ed.).* St. Louis, MO: Elsevier Mosby, Inc.

Wagenfeld, A. & Kaldenberg, J. (2005). *Foundations of Pediatric Practice for the Occupational Therapy Assistant.* Thorofare, NJ: SLACK, Inc.

Watson, D.E. & Wilson, S.A. (2003). *Task Analysis: An Individual and Population Approach (2nd ed.).* Bethesda, MD: AOTA Press.

Zoltan, B. (2007). *Vision, Perception, and Cognition: A Manual for the Evaluation and Treatment of the Adult with Acquired Brain Injury (4th ed.).* Thorofare, NJ: SLACK, Inc.

---

*   *References cited during introductory chapter of this study guide. These references should not be viewed as examination item references.*

Appendix C - Abbreviations used on the Certification Examination

The following is a list of abbreviations (acronyms) that are to be used in examination items:

ADA	=	The Americans with Disabilities Act
ADL	=	Activities of Daily Living (not ADLs or ADL's)
AIDS	=	Acquired Immune Deficiency Syndrome
BADL	=	Basic Activities of Daily Living
COPD	=	Chronic Obstructive Pulmonary Disease
COTA	=	CERTIFIED OCCUPATIONAL THERAPY ASSISTANT COTA®
CPR	=	Cardiopulmonary Resuscitation
CVA	=	Cerebrovascular Accident
DIP	=	Distal Interphalangeal*
DSM IV	=	Diagnostic and Statistical Manual of Mental Disorders - 4th Ed.
HIPAA	=	Health Information Portability and Accountability Act
HIV	=	Human Immunodeficiency Virus
IADL	=	Instrumental Activities of Daily Living
IEP	=	Individual Education Program
MCP	=	Metacarpophalangeal
MP	=	Metacarpophalangeal
NDT	=	Neuro-Developmental Treatment
OTR	=	OCCUPATIONAL THERAPIST REGISTERED OTR®
PADL	=	Personal Activities of Daily Living
PIP	=	Proximal Interphalangeal*
ROM	=	Range of Motion
SCI	=	Spinal cord injury
SOAP	=	Subjective, Objective, Assessment, Plan Components of the Problem-Oriented Medical Record
TBI	=	Traumatic Brain Injury
TTY/TDD	=	Teletypewriter/telecommunication device for the deaf

*Must be followed by the word "joint"

Diagnoses/Conditions

ADHD
Adjustment disorders
Alcohol/substance abuse
Amyotrophic Lateral Sclerosis
Alzheimer's Disease
Amputation/Prostheses
Anxiety disorders
Aphasia
Apraxia
Arthritis/Collagen Injury
Ataxia/Incoordination
Autism
Autonomic Dysreflexia
Back Pain
Balance
Bipolar disorders
Blood pressure/hypertension
Body scheme/apraxia/neglect
Burns
Cardiopulmonary disease
COPD
Ischemia
Respiratory
Carpal tunnel
Cognitive dysfunction
Cerebral Palsy
Complex Regional Pain Syndrome
Cumulative trauma disorders
    DeQuervain's Disease
    Carpal Tunnel Syndrome
    Lateral Epicondylitis
    Cubital Tunnel Syndrome
CVA/Hemiplegia
Death/Dying/Hospice
Decubitis Ulcers
Deep Vein Thrombosis
Dementia/Alzheimer's/Memory
Depression
Desensitization

Developmental Disorders
    Autism
    Asperger's
    Developmental Delay
    Down Syndrome
Diabetes
Distractibility/Concentration
Domestic violence/Abuse—Child/Spousal/
    Elder
Dysphagia/Swallow
Dyspraxia
Eating disorders
Edema
Encephalopathy
Falls
Fetal Alcohol Syndrome
Fibromyalgia
Figure ground
Flexibility/flexion
Fractures
Grasp/grip
Guillain Barré
Hand Injury
Hemiplegia/hemiparesis
Heterotropic Ossification
Hip/Knee/Joint replacement
HIV/AIDS
Hypertonia/spasticity
Hypotonicity/flaccidity
Joints/MCP/PIP
Learning disabilities
Muscular Dystrophy
Medications/Side Effects
Motor skills/planning/control
Motor skills/planning/control
Mental Retardation
Multiple Sclerosis
Muscle tone
Neurodevelopmental Treatment (NDT)

Nerve injuries/Peripheral Neuropathy
Normal Child Development
Oral/Tongue
OCD
Osteoporosis
Pain
Paralysis
Parkinson's/tremors
Perception
Perserveration
Personality disorder
Pervasive Developmental Disorder
Positioning/Trunk control
Post-polio Syndrome
Post Traumatic Stress Disorder
Postural Hypotension
Reading disorders
Reflexes
ATNR
STNR
Labyrinthine
Head Righting
ROM/PROM
Schizophrenia
SCI
      Paraplegia
      Tetraplegia
      Quadriplegia
Sensation
Sensory Integrative Disorders
Sequencing
Scar Remodeling—
Hypertrophic scar
Spasticity
Spina Bifida
Suicidal Ideation
Tactile defensiveness
Tardive Dyskinesia
TBI
Tenosynovitis/deQuervain's
Tonic bite
Vision impairments
      Low Vision
Macular degeneration
Homonymous hemianopsia
Work-related injuries

Interventions/Treatments/Equipment

Activities of Daily Living (ADL)
Age-appropriate/Graded activity
Augmentative Communication
Assessment tools
Assistive/Adaptive Environment
Assistive Devices
Adaptiveutensils Assistive technology
Behavior Modification
Biomechanical
Body Mechanics
Chaining
Forward chaining
Backward chaining
Client-Centered Approaches
Cognitive–Perceptual Retraining
Community Integration
Community Referrals
Compensatory Techniques
Coping Strategies
Desensitization
Discharge Planning
Energy Conservation
Endurance/strength/exercise
Environmental Modification
Ergonomics
Goal-Setting
Graded activities
Group dynamics
Home program education
Joint Protection
Lifestyle redesign
Muscle testing
Patient Education
Positioning
Pressure garments
Purposeful Activity
Range of Motion Exercises
Role play
Safety
Universal Precautions
Sanitation
Sensory Reeducation
Splint Fabrication/Modification
Strengthening Exercises

Appendices

D

Transfer Training/Education
Wheelchair Assessment/Modification
Wheelchair/Functional Mobility
Work Hardening/Functional Capacity
Work Simplification

Service Components

Communication skills
Confidentiality
Conflict of Interest
Cultural Sensitivity/Diversity
    Culturally responsive care
COTA/OTR roles & responsibilities
CQI/Performance improvement
Discharge Planning/Documentation Methods
Documentation Method/Responsibilities
Evaluation/Reevaluation
Frames of Reference / Models of Practice
Informed consent
Insurance authorization/reimbursement
Interviewing skills/methods
Multidisciplinary Team Process
    Listening
Negotiating
Conflict resolution
    Roles & responsibilities
Professional Liability
Program evaluation
Promoting the Profession
Refusal of service
Research methods
Reliability
Validity
Research design
Resource Management
    Time
Equipment
Supplies
Screening
Service Collaboration
Service Competencies
Strategic planning/goals

Settings/Situations

Acute Care Hospital
Adult Daycare Center
ADA
Architectural/Environmental barriers
Assisted Living Facilities
Automobile
Bathing/Bathroom
Classroom
Clinic
Cooking
Community-based
Consultant
Daycare Facility
Dressing
Eating/Dining
Grooming/hygiene
Groups—Inpatient/Outpatient
Group Home
Home-based
IDEA
Independence
Inpatient Rehab Facility
Interests
Job elements
Leisure
Long-term care facility
Occupation
Playground
Play/leisure activities
Prison/Confinement Facility
School-based
Skilled Nursing Facility
Toileting
Treatments—New/Unfamiliar
Volunteers
Wellness programs
Workplace
Writing/prewriting

01   GATHER INFORMATION AND FORMULATE CONCLUSIONS REGARDING THE CLIENT'S NEEDS AND PRIORITIES TO DEVELOP A CLIENT-CENTERED INTERVENTION PLAN

01.01   *Gather information on an ongoing basis using appropriate tools, procedures, and protocols in order to identify factors that impact participation in occupation.*

01.01.01	Information gathering processes and procedures (e.g., observation, interview, client records, checklists)
01.01.02	Procedures and protocols for standardized tests
01.01.03	Normal development and function across the lifespan
01.01.04	Expected patterns/progressions associated with conditions that limit occupational performance
01.01.05	Performance patterns (e.g., habits, routines, roles, values) of the client
01.01.06	Client contexts (cultural, physical, social, personal, spiritual, temporal, and virtual)
01.01.07	Activity demands
01.01.08	Appropriate responses to unexpected occurrences during the information gathering process

01.02   *Contribute comprehensive information regarding the impact of current condition(s) and context(s) on the client's occupational performance in order to assist the OTR in formulating an intervention plan.*

01.02.01	Therapeutic use of occupations and activities across the lifespan
01.02.02	Life skills relevant to culture roles, habits, and routines, and current abilities (e.g., home management, social skills, vocational skills)
01.02.03	Activity analysis methods related to client roles, habits and routines, and current abilities
01.02.04	Components of an intervention plan
01.02.05	Levels of service provision
01.02.06	Impact of the environment on the client's occupational performance
01.02.07	Internal and external influences on occupational performance (e.g., disability, environment, context, medication)
01.02.08	Clinical reasoning strategies and approaches

01.03   *Collaborate with the OTR, client, and relevant others using a team approach in order to prioritize client centered goals throughout the continuum of care, guided by evidence and the principles of best practice.*

01.03.01	Team roles, responsibilities, and care coordination
01.03.02	Collaborative, client-centered strategies for setting goals based on expected outcomes
01.03.03	Methods and techniques for promoting carry-over of intervention within the transitional environment, home, work, school, or community
01.03.04	Frequency and duration of intervention needed to reach goals
01.03.05	Discharge planning procedures
01.03.06	Transitional services

01.04 *Provide information to the OTR regarding the need for referral to other professionals or services in order to facilitate comprehensive, quality care.*

01.04.01	Potential referral sources and processes
01.04.02	Service delivery models
01.04.03	Role delineation and the contributions of other services providers
01.04.04	Appropriate community resources, funding, reimbursement, and/or payment sources

02   SELECT AND IMPLEMENT EVIDENCE-BASED INTERVENTIONS TO SUPPORT PARTICIPATION IN AREAS OF OCCUPATION (e.g., ADL, EDUCATION, WORK, PLAY, LEISURE, AND SOCIAL PARTICIPATION) THROUGHOUT THE CONTINUUM OF CARE

02.01 *Implement the treatment plan by using critical reasoning to select interventions and approaches consistent with general medical, neurological, and musculoskeletal conditions and client needs in order to achieve functional outcomes within areas of occupation.*

02.01.01	Impact of general medical, neurological, and musculoskeletal conditions on areas of occupation (e.g., ADL, work, leisure, social participation, education, play)
02.01.02	Activities to enhance performance in areas of occupation
02.01.03	Compensatory strategies and techniques for minimizing the impact of disease process and/or condition on occupational performance (e.g., joint protection, work simplification, and energy conservation, occupational modification)
02.01.04	Biomechanical strategies and techniques that impact strength, motion, and endurance (e.g., ROM and strengthening exercise, wound care, edema control principles and techniques)
02.01.05	Remedial and preventive strategies and techniques specific to general medical conditions (e.g., scar management, pressure-relief techniques, positioning, infection control, standard precautions) for developing or restoring a skill or ability
02.01.06	Facilitation and handling principles and techniques for improving functional performance consistent with general medical, neurological, and/or musculoskeletal conditions
02.01.07	Safe and effective administration of superficial thermal and mechanical physical agent modalities as an adjunct to participation in activities
02.01.08	Methods for selecting, designing, fabricating and modifying common splints, consistent with general medical, neurological, and/or musculoskeletal conditions
02.01.09	Methods for selecting, designing, fabricating, and/or modifying adaptive equipment and assistive devices consistent with general medical, neurological, and/or musculoskeletal conditions
02.01.10	Interventions for facilitating chewing and swallowing specific to general medical conditions
02.01.11	Positioning and physical transfer techniques consistent with activity demands, client skills, and abilities
02.01.12	Neurobehavioral techniques for skill development consistent with general medical, neurological, and/or musculoskeletal conditions (e.g., visual scanning, hand-over-hand techniques, visual cueing, verbal prompting)

02.02 *Implement the treatment plan by using critical reasoning to select interventions and approaches consistent with developmental level, pediatric conditions, and/or congenital anomalies and client needs in order to achieve functional outcomes within areas of occupation.*

02.02.01	Impact of developmental level, pediatric conditions, and/or congenital anomalies on areas of occupation (e.g., ADL, education, leisure, play, social participation)
02.02.02	Normal development for task accomplishment
02.02.03	Facilitation and handling principles and techniques consistent with developmental level, pediatric conditions, and/or congenital anomalies
02.02.04	Activities to promote development in areas of occupation
02.02.05	Visual and perceptual skill development skills
02.02.06	Sensory integrative interventions and sensory modulation techniques
02.02.07	Remedial, compensatory, and preventive techniques specific to developmental level, pediatric conditions, and/or congenital anomalies (e.g., positioning, standard precautions)
02.02.08	Methods for selecting, designing, fabricating and modifying common splints, consistent with developmental level, pediatric conditions, and/or congenital anomalies
02.02.09	Methods for selecting, designing, fabricating, and/or modifying adaptive equipment and assistive devices consistent with developmental level, pediatric conditions, and/or congenital anomalies
02.02.10	Behavior management techniques appropriate to developmental level.
02.02.11	Protocol-based interventions for facilitating chewing and swallowing specific to developmental level, pediatric conditions, and/or congenital anomalies
02.02.12	Positioning and physical transfer techniques consistent with developmental levels and activity demands
02.02.13	Neurobehavioral techniques for skill acquisition consistent with developmental level, pediatric conditions, and/or congenital anomalies

02.03 *Implement the treatment plan by using critical reasoning to select interventions and approaches consistent with psychosocial and cognitive abilities, and client needs in order to achieve functional outcomes within areas of occupation.*

02.03.01	Impact of psychosocial and cognitive abilities on areas of occupation (e.g., ADL, education, leisure, play, social participation)
02.03.02	Methods and techniques for facilitating groups appropriate to participants' psychosocial and cognitive abilities
02.03.03	Activities for enhancing skills within areas of occupation
02.03.04	Techniques for responding in a therapeutic manner to the needs of a client and/ or caregiver during psychosocial interventions
02.03.05	Intervention strategies appropriate for psychosocial and cognitive models of practice (e.g., coping skills, stress management, biofeedback, relaxation, cognitive behavioral therapy)
02.03.06	Remedial, compensatory, and preventive techniques consistent with psychosocial and cognitive status (e.g., problem solving worksheets, medication management, memory aids, falls prevention)
02.03.07	Methods for selecting, designing, fabricating, and/or modifying adaptive equipment or assistive devices consistent with psychosocial and/or cognitive abilities

02.04 *Maximize accessibility to and mobility within a client's contexts by recommending environmental modifications in order to optimize occupational performance and/or enhance quality of life.*

02.04.01	Impact of the environment on occupational performance
02.04.02	Methods for environmental modification within contexts (e.g., transitional environments, home, work, school, community)
02.04.03	Accessibility concerns and barriers (e.g., ADA guidelines)
02.04.04	Community transport alternatives
02.04.05	Types and functions of seating and mobility systems, durable medical equipment, environmental modifications, and/or assistive technology
02.04.06	Methods for teaching individuals about the safe use and proper care of seating and mobility systems, durable medical equipment, and assistive technology within a variety of contexts
02.04.07	Product information related to environmental adaptations.
02.04.08	Ergonomic principles and universal design
02.04.09	Methods of adapting the home and/or community environment

02.05 *Modify intervention methods and techniques based on the client's needs and responses in order to promote occupational performance.*

02.05.01	Physical, psychological, and social responses requiring modification of the intervention methods and techniques
02.05.02	Methods for adjusting intervention techniques in response to variances from anticipated outcomes
02.05.03	Methods of adapting the intervention environment based on medical status and behavioral responses to maximize participation in areas of occupation
02.05.04	Methods for grading an intervention activity based on expected progress and/or unexpected physical responses
02.05.05	Methods for responding appropriately to unexpected occurrences during intervention

02.06 *Apply the principles of health promotion, wellness, prevention, and/or educational programming based on client and community needs in order to serve as a resource for occupation based program activities.*

02.06.01	Participation in meaningful occupations and its relationship to health well being, and life satisfaction
02.06.02	Health promotion and wellness programming for various populations

03 UPHOLD PROFESSIONAL STANDARDS AND RESPONSIBILITIES TO PROMOTE QUALITY IN PRACTICE

03.01 *Maintaining ongoing competence by participating in professional development activities in order to provide effective services and promote quality care.*

03.01.01	Professional development activities
03.01.02	NBCOT certification renewal policies
03.01.03	Methods of reviewing and applying professional literature to practice

03.02 *Upholding professional standards by participating in continuous quality improvement activities and complying with safety regulations, laws, ethical codes, facility policies and procedures, and guidelines governing OT practice in order to protect the public interest*

03.02.01	Policies, procedures, and guidelines related to service provision
03.02.02	Ethical decision making
03.02.03	NBCOT code of conduct
03.02.04	Client confidentiality regulations (e.g., HIPAA)
03.02.05	State and federal laws governing OT practice
03.02.06	Methods for incorporating federally mandated guidelines into intervention plans
03.02.07	Safety procedures and risk management techniques
03.02.08	Accrediting bodies and their requirements
03.02.09	Standards/scope of practice for OT
03.02.10	Quality improvement processes and procedures (includes participation in program evaluation and outcomes measures)

03.03 *Document occupational therapy services using established guidelines in order to verify accountability and to meet the requirements of practice settings, accrediting bodies, regulatory agencies, and/or funding sources.*

03.03.01	Types, formats, and purposes of documentation
03.03.02	Reimbursement systems and regulatory requirements for documentation

03.04 *Articulate how occupational therapy contributes to beneficial outcomes for clients and relevant others based on evidence in order to promote quality care.*

03.04.01	Roles and responsibilities of certified OT practitioners
03.04.02	Effective communication methods and strategies
03.04.03	Components and organization of effective presentations

03.05 *Supervise occupational therapy students, paraprofessionals, and volunteers in accordance with professional guidelines and applicable regulations in order to support the delivery of appropriate occupational therapy services.*

03.05.01	Clinical fieldwork education
03.05.02	Regulatory requirements and professional standards for supervision
03.05.03	OTR and COTA role delineation